PATHOLOGY
PICTURE TESTS

Alan Stevens MBBS FRC Path
Senior Lecturer in Histopathology, University of Nottingham Medical School
Honorary Consultant Histopathologist to Queen's Medical Centre
University Hospital NHS Trust, Nottingham, UK

James Lowe BMedSci BMBS DM MRCPath
Reader in Pathology, University of Nottingham Medical School
Honorary Consultant Neuropathologist to Queen's Medical Centre
University Hospital NHS Trust, Nottingham, UK

Gillian Kirk MB ChB
Formerly Registrar in Histopathology
Queen's Medical Centre
University Hospital NHS Trust, Nottingham, UK

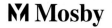

M Mosby

London Baltimore Bogotá Boston Buenos Aires Caracàs Carlsbad, CA Chicago Madrid Mexico City
Milan Naples, FL New York Philadelphia St. Louis Sydney Tokyo Toronto Wiesbaden

Project Manager:	Dave Burin
Developmental Editor:	Rachael Miller
Illustration:	Lynda Payne
Cover Design:	Pete Wilder
Production:	Jane Tozer
Publisher:	Fiona Foley

Published in 1995 by Mosby, an imprint of Times Mirror International Publishers Limited

Printed by Grafos SA Arte sobre papel, Barcelona, Spain

ISBN 0 7234 2192 7

For full details of all Times Mirror International Publishers Limited titles, please write to Times Mirror International Publishers Limited, Lynton House, 7–12 Tavistock Square, London WC1H 9LB, England.

A CIP catalogue record for this book is available from the British Library.

Library of Congress Cataloging-in-Publication Data has been applied for.

PREFACE

Students enjoy looking at pictures. A carefully selected photograph or a well-drawn diagram is easier to assimilate than written text, and is easier to recall and reproduce under examination conditions. The combination of a clear illustration with a simple written description greatly increases students understanding of a topic. For this reason , our textbook *Pathology*, published by Mosby, is lavishly illustrated with full-colour photographs and superbly drawn diagrams. *Pathology Picture Tests* is derived from this parent book and is intended as a feedback and revision aid, so that students can assess the extent or limitations of their understanding. Additional material related to clinical aspects of disease has been included to emphasise the central role of pathology in medicine. Illustrations taken from *Pathology* are used as the focus for questions dealing with important aspects of the subject. Brief answers to these questions are given together with page references to the parent book for more detailed information.

We wish to thank Fiona Foley and Rachael Miller who, on behalf of Mosby, subsidised several working lunches during the production of *Pathology Picture Tests*.

AS
JL
GK

CONTENTS

	Pages
Questions	**5–87**
Cellular Adaptations to Disease	5–6
Cell Injury and Death	7–10
Neoplasia	10–13
Tissue Responses to Damage	14–20
Developmental and Genetic Factors in Disease	21–23
Immune, Infective, Environmental, and Nutritional Factors in Disease	24–25
Blood Circulatory System	26–32
The Respiratory System	33–37
Oral and ENT Pathology	38–40
Alimentary Tract	41–45
Liver, Biliary Tract, and Pancreas	46–50
Lymphoid and Haemopoietic Tissues	51–53
Endocrine System	54–57
Urinary System	58–65
Male Genital System	66–68
Gynaecological and Obstetric Pathology	69–72
Breast Disease	73–75
Nervous System and Muscle	76–82
Dermatopathology	83
Orthopaedic and Rheumatological Pathology	84–87
Answers	**89–128**

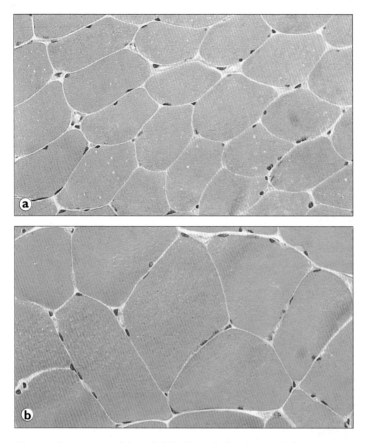

Photomicrographs (a) and (b) show skeletal muscle in transverse section at the same magnification. Both are normal but (b) shows a common adaptive process.

Q1. What is the adaptive process in (b)?

Q2. What is the likely cause of this adaptive change?

Q3. Fill in the missing words:

.... (i)............ is an increase in the size of existing cells accompanied by an increase in their functional capacity.

.... (ii)........... is an increase in the number of cells in a tissue caused by increased cell division.

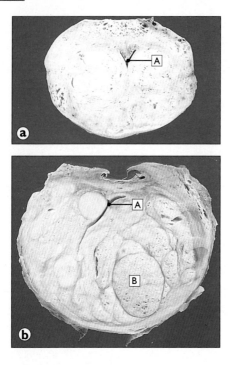

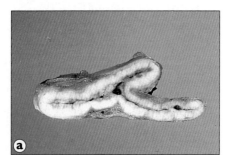

Figure (a) shows a slice through a normal prostate gland, and Figure (b) a slice through an abnormal prostate at the same magnification.

Q4. What is the structure labelled **A** in both pictures?

Q5. What is the disease process in (b)?

Q6. What is the structure labelled **B**?

Q7. What symptoms does this disease process produce, what physical signs, and what are the long-term complications?

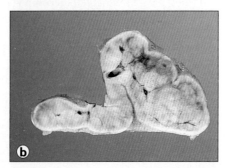

Figures (a) and (b) show slices of adrenal glands removed at autopsy: (a) from a patient with long-standing crippling rheumatoid arthritis; (b) from a normal patient.

Q8. What pathological process does (a) show?

Q9. In view of the patient's history, what do you think is the most likely cause and what is its mechanism?

Q10. What precautions must be taken with such patients and why?

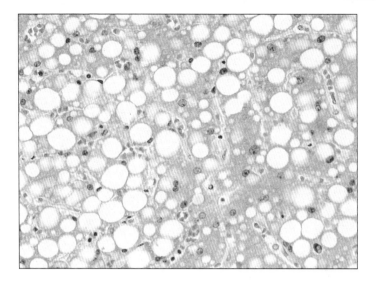

This micrograph of liver shows a particular pattern of cytological abnormality.

Q11. The abnormality in the cytoplasm is the presence of numerous round vacuoles. What do they contain and what is the name of this abnormality?

Q12. What are the four main metabolic causes for this change?

Q13. This tissue was obtained in life by biopsying the organ of a 57-year-old bar owner. What is the likely cause in this case, and what is its most important complication?

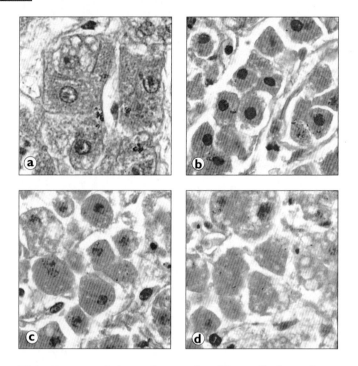

This sequence of photomicrographs of liver cells shows the changes which can be seen in cells undergoing necrosis: namely, karyolysis, cytoplasmic vacuolation, karyorrhexis and pyknosis.

Q14. Match each of the above steps to a photograph.

Q15. What are the characteristic features of each step?

Q16. What is the correct sequence?

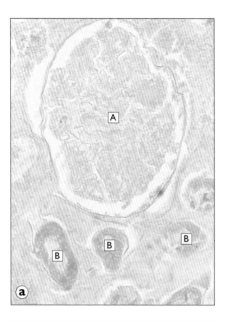

Photomicrographs (a) and (b) show colliquative and coagulative patterns of necrosis.

Q17. Which is which?

Q18. Which organ do you think is involved in the coagulative necrosis?

Q19. Which organ is most likely to be involved in the colliquative necrosis?

Q20. Which general process has led to necrosis in these two organs?

Q21. What is the likely outcome of these two patterns of necrosis?

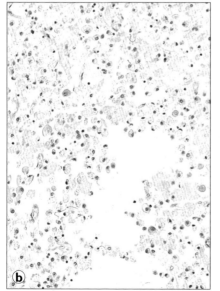

Cell damaged	Enzyme elevated in blood
A	Creatine kinase (MB isoform) Aspartate transaminase (AST) Lactate dehydrogenase (LDH-1)
Hepatocyte	Alanine transaminase (ALT)
Striated muscle	Creatine kinase (MM isoform)
Exocrine pancreas	**B**

Q22. This table illustrates the release of enzymes into the blood following cell or tissue damage. Fill in the missing words at **A** and **B**.

Q23. A 45-year-old business man returns from a business conference in Amsterdam, and is admitted with severe upper abdominal pain of 4 hours' duration. He is overweight, a smoker and a heavy social drinker. Which of the above enzymes would you measure and why?

Q24. In suspected myocardial infarction, blood levels of enzyme are measured sequentially over 3 days. Why?

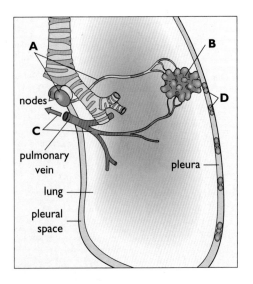

This diagram shows the 4 main patterns of spread of a malignant tumour, here exemplified by carcinoma of the lung.

Q25. Name the types of spread in **A**, **B**, **C**, and **D**.

Q26. In the case of carcinoma of the bronchus, which are the most common organs in which metastases occur due to spread of tumour by method **C**?

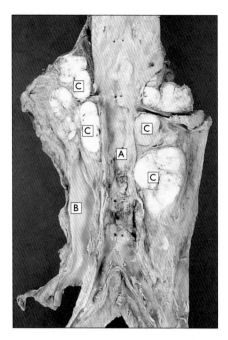

Q27. In this photograph of a gross specimen, identify the structures labelled **A**, **B** and **C**.

Q28. What abnormality does **A** show?

Q29. What abnormality is present in **C**?

Q30. What are the possibilities to explain the abnormalities in **C**?

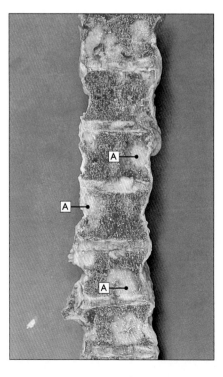

Q31. What is this structure removed at post-mortem?

Q32. What are the lesions labelled **A**?

Q33. What conditions affecting what other organs can lead to this?

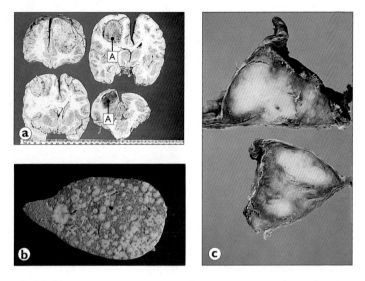

These three organs were removed at post-mortem from the same patient, a man aged 66. They are (a) brain, (b) liver and (c) adrenal.

Q34. Describe what each shows macroscopically.

Q35. What disease process has produced the lesions?

Q36. What is the most likely unifying diagnosis in this case, and what other organ would you therefore like to examine?

Q37. What is the usual cause for the appearance seen in (b)?

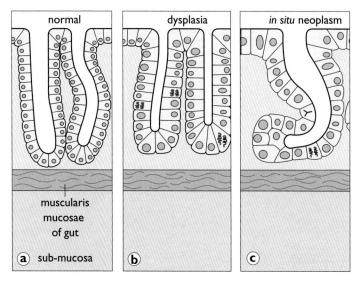

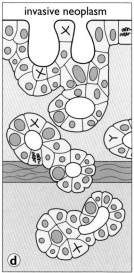

This sequence of diagrams shows the progression from normal epithelium, through dysplastic epithelium, to carcinoma *in situ* and finally invasive carcinoma, exemplified by a site in the alimentary tract—for example, the gastric mucosa—associated with long-standing chronic gastritis.

Q38. Where else in the alimentary tract may this sequence occur and in what circumstances?

Q39. Name two other non-alimentary sites where this sequence of progressive changes commonly occurs.

Q40. Is it possible to prevent the progression to invasive cancer?

Q41. How may dysplasia be diagnosed?

Tumour marker	Tumour
Alpha fetoprotein (AFP)	Hepatocellular carcinoma Germ cell tumours
Human chorionic gonadotrophin (HCG)	**A**
Acid phosphatase	**B**
Carcinoembryonic antigen (CEA)	Gastrointestinal tract neoplasia
Hormone products	**C**

This table shows some of the tumour markers used in diagnosis.

Q42. Fill in the missing words at **A**, **B** and **C**.

Q43. How are these tumour markers sampled?

Q44. Other than assisting in the initial diagnosis of tumour type, what other reasons are there for continued monitoring of tumour marker levels such as HCG?

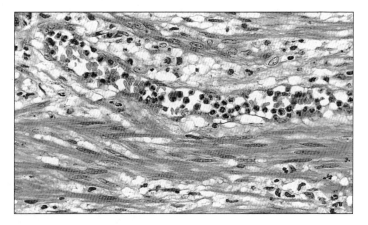

This photomicrograph shows a blood vessel in an early stage of the acute inflammatory reaction.

Q45. What is happening in the blood vessel lumen?

Q46. What is the major cell type accumulating?

Q47. What happens next?

Q48. What is the single most common outcome of an acute inflammatory reaction to an area of tissue damage?

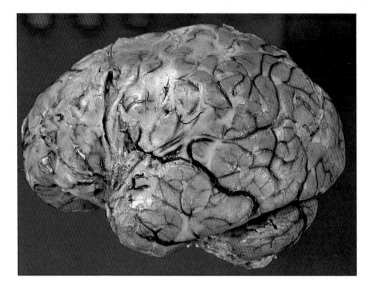

This photograph shows the brain of a young child who was admitted in a coma following a short history of malaise, fever and drowsiness.

Q49. What are the dark lines coursing over the surface of the brain?

Q50. What is the creamy material spread over the frontal and parietal cortex?

Q51. What is the disease and what is the most likely cause in this case?

Q52. What is the most important laboratory investigation in patients with this disease?

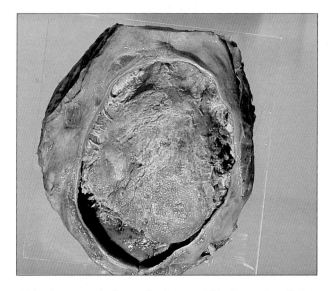

This photograph shows the heart within its pericardial sac, a window having been cut in the parietal pericardium to expose the visceral pericardium overlying the heart.

Q53. What is wrong with the visceral pericardium to produce the thick rough appearance?

Q54. How does this pattern of inflammatory reaction differ from that seen over the brain in **Q49–52**? Why is there a difference?

Q55. What is the most likely cause of this change and how may it be manifest on clinical examination?

Q56. What is the most likely outcome of the pericardial changes if the patient survives?

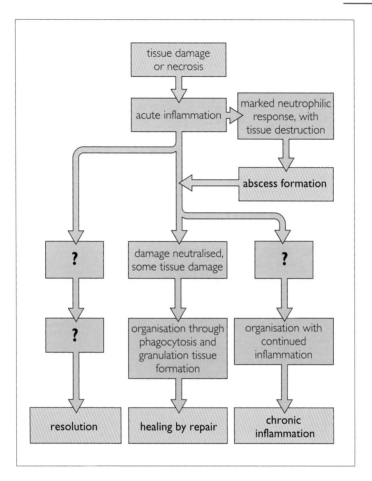

This flow chart shows the possible outcomes of an area of tissue damage or necrosis.

Q57. What factors allow healing by resolution?

Q58. What factors lead to a state of chronic inflammation?

Q59. Which of the three outcomes (resolution, healing by repair or chronic inflammation) is the most common?

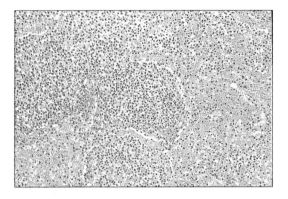

This photomicrograph shows a histological section of the lung alveoli in a patient who died after a 4-day history of fever, cough, increasing breathlessness and stabbing chest pain on the right lower side. At post-mortem examination the right lower lobe was solid and airless, with a uniform brown-grey colour.

Q60. What do the alveoli contain? What is the diagnosis and likely cause?

Q61. If the patient had survived what would have happened to the material in the alveoli, and how would normal function of the affected lobe have been restored?

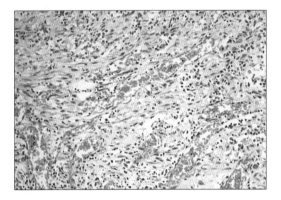

This photomicrograph shows highly vascular tissue, largely composed of distended blood-filled new capillaries, taken from the area of the floor of a chronic peptic ulcer immediately beneath the necrotic ulcer slough.

Q62. What is this tissue called?

Q63. What are the steps by which this temporary tissue converts into a strong fibrous scar?

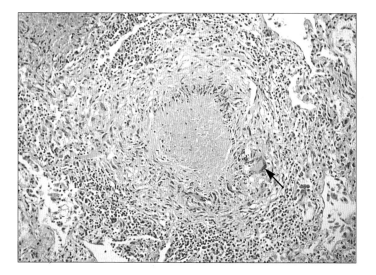

This photomicrograph shows the histology of one of many minute nodular lesions from the lung of an elderly homeless man who was found dead in a bus shelter one morning after a very cold night. There was also a large cavitating abscess in the right upper pole of the lung, and multiple pinhead-size white nodules in the spleen, liver and kidney. The photomicrograph shows a particular type of chronic inflammation.

Q64. What is the name given to this pattern of chronic inflammation?

Q65. What is the most likely cause in this case?

Q66. What is the name given to the amorphous pink material in the centre and the multinucleate giant cell (arrowed) at the edge of the lesion?

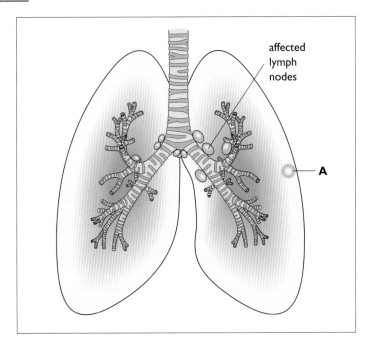

This artwork illustrates the pattern of involvement of the lung in primary-type pulmonary tuberculosis; the areas affected by tuberculosis are coloured yellow.

Q67. What is the name given to the lesion labelled **A**?

Q68. The combination of **A** and involved regional lymph nodes is called what?

Q69. What would be the outcome of this infection in a normal healthy well-nourished, non-immunosuppressed child?

Q70. What would be the possible outcomes in a malnourished or immunosuppressed child?

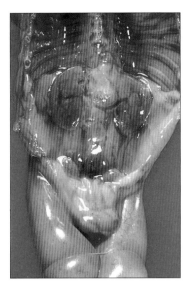

This photograph, taken from a stillborn fetus, shows complete failure of development of the kidneys; the two organs visible at the site of the kidneys are large fetal adrenal glands.

Q71. What is the name given to complete failure of organ development as seen here?

Q72. What is the name of the syndrome associated with complete failure of kidney development?

Q73. What feature of the pregnancy is apparent when the fetus has complete failure of development of kidneys, and why?

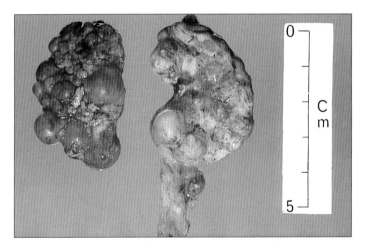

This photomicrograph shows kidneys removed at post-mortem from an infant which died shortly after birth without ever passing urine. The mother had oligohydramnios. The kidneys are replaced by a disorganised mass of cysts.

Q74. This is an example of abnormal tissue organisation. What name is given to this process?

Q75. Why did the infant pass no urine?

Q76. Why did the mother have oligohydramnios?

Q77. Does this process always affect all of both kidneys?

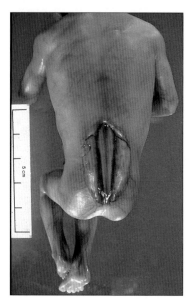

This photograph of a stillborn fetus shows a common and important congenital malformation.

Q78. What is it called, and how has it arisen?

Q79. With what intracranial abnormality is it frequently associated?

Q80. How may this condition be diagnosed *in utero*?

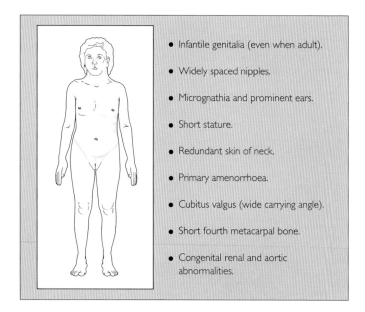

- Infantile genitalia (even when adult).

- Widely spaced nipples.

- Micrognathia and prominent ears.

- Short stature.

- Redundant skin of neck.

- Primary amenorrhoea.

- Cubitus valgus (wide carrying angle).

- Short fourth metacarpal bone.

- Congenital renal and aortic abnormalities.

Q81. What syndrome is illustrated in the above diagram?

Q82. What is the name commonly given to the presence of the redundant skin at the neck?

Q83. What is the chromosomal make-up in the non-mosaic form of this syndrome, and how may it arise?

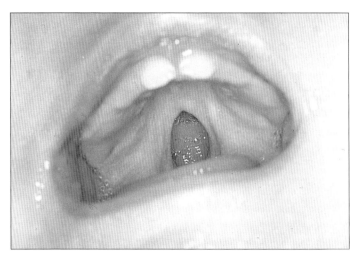

Q84. What is this common congenital malformation?

Q85. What other structural congenital abnormality is this often associated with?

Q86. What type of embryological maldevelopment pattern is this an example of?

Q87. What are the main problems encountered by a patient with this abnormality and can they be treated?

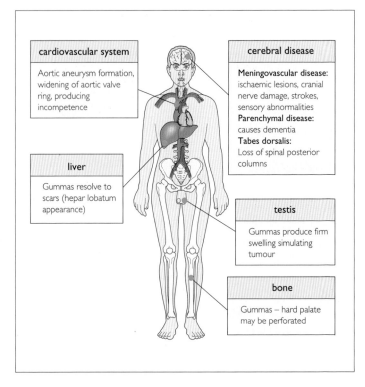

Q88. The above artwork shows the widespread late manifestations of what disease?

Q89. What is the causative organism?

Q90. What is a gumma?

Q91. What is the name given to the primary lesion in this illness?

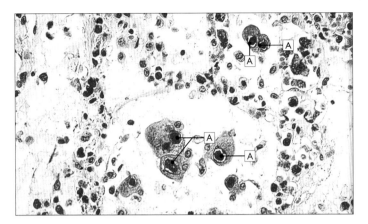

This photomicrograph shows the histology of the lung in a young woman who died with respiratory problems some time after a renal transplant.

Q92. What are the structures labelled **A**?

Q93. What is the most likely causative organism in this case?

Q94. Why is the history of renal transplantation important?

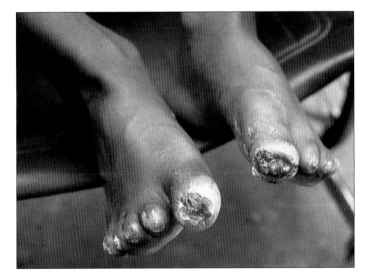

This photograph is from a Himalayan mountain guide.

Q95. What is the disease?

Q96. What is the mechanism?

Q97. What other parts of the anatomy may be involved?

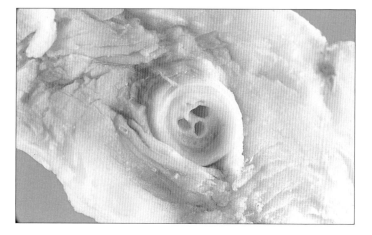

This photograph shows an abnormal coronary artery cut in transverse section, surrounded by epicardial fat.

Q98. What abnormality does the coronary artery show?

Q99. What sequence of events has led to this appearance?

Q100. What would this patient's heart show at post-mortem examination?

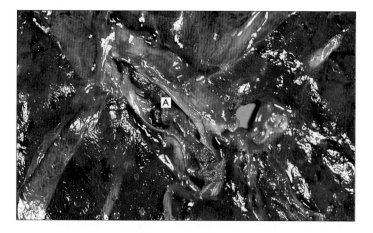

This photograph taken at post-mortem examination shows an example of pulmonary thromboembolism (**A**).

Q101. Is the thrombus in a major pulmonary artery or vein?

Q102. What is the most likely source of the embolic material?

Q103. By what route did the embolic material get into this pulmonary vessel?

Q104. What is the most likely outcome of a pulmonary embolism of this size?

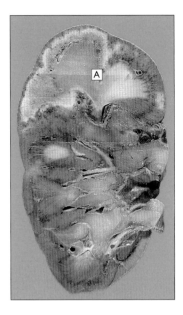

This kidney was taken from a 64-year-old man with a history of angina and a recent myocardial infarct. Shortly before his death he developed a dense right hemiplegia and loin pain.

Q105. What is the lesion at the upper pole (**A**)?

Q106. Bearing in mind the history, what is the most likely cause?

Q107. What will the pale area show under the microscope?

Q108. What is the likely cause of his hemiplegia?

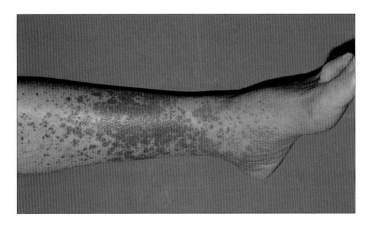

The left leg of a woman aged 43, on treatment for rheumatoid arthritis, is shown. The right leg showed identical changes, and there was a similar but less severe rash on the thighs.

Q109. What is the name given to this type of skin rash?

Q110. What is the cause of the confluent small red blotches?

Q111. What factors in the history may be significant in deducing the cause?

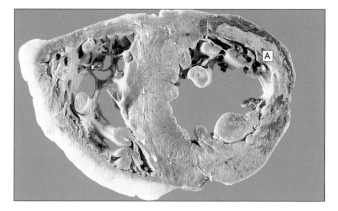

This is a transverse section of the right and left ventricles from a heart removed at post-mortem examination from a man aged 58 with a history of hypertension, found dead at home. His daughter said that he had complained of chest pain and breathlessness for some days.

Q112. What is the lesion labelled **A** in the lateral wall of the left ventricle?

Q113. How long has it been present?

Q114. Bearing in mind the location of the lesion, what other abnormality would the heart probably show?

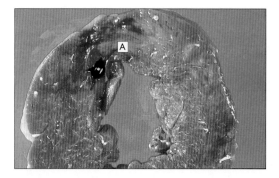

This slice across the left ventricle was from a woman aged 72 who collapsed and died while walking in the street. At post-mortem examination, her pericardial cavity was filled with blood.

Q115. What name is given to the condition where the pericardial cavity is filled with blood?

Q116. What are the effects of sudden distension of the pericardial cavity with blood?

Q117. What is the most likely cause in the case shown above?

Q118. What is the other common spontaneous cause?

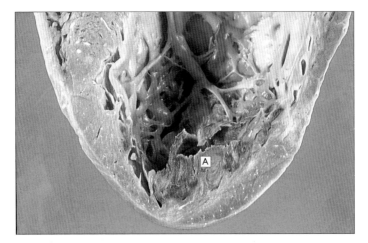

This photograph shows a vertical slice through the apex of the left ventricle taken at post-mortem examination in a 75-year-old man who died shortly after onset of a dense right hemiplegia.

Q119. What is lesion **A**, and how has it formed?

Q120. This is an important early complication of myocardial infarction. What are the others?

Q121. Why did the patient have a stroke?

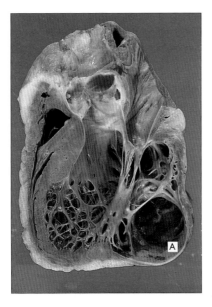

This photograph shows the heart removed at post-mortem examination from an elderly man with intractable left heart failure. It shows an important long-term complication of myocardial infarction.

Q122. What is the structural abnormality labelled **A** and how has it arisen?

Q123. What are the other long-term complications of myocardial infarction?

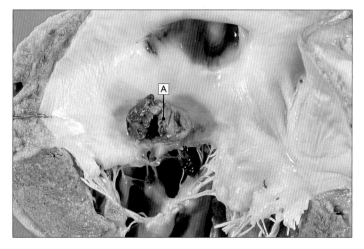

Q124. What is the structure labelled **A** on this mitral valve leaflet?
Q125. Of what is it composed?
Q126. What circumstances predispose to this condition?
Q127. What are the complications?

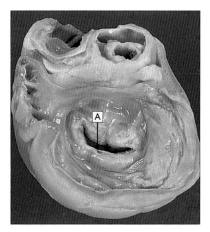

This photograph shows the floor of the left atrium viewed from above, with the mitral valve orifice reduced to a narrow slit (**A**).

Q128. What is the disease and how has the deformity of the mitral valve orifice been produced?

Q129. What was the patient's original illness which has led to this late complication?

Q130. What are the haemodynamic consequences of this abnormality?

Q131. Which other valve may be involved in this disease process?

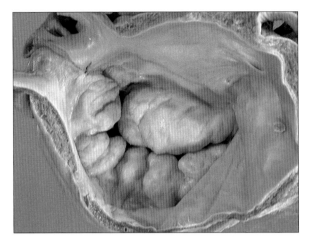

This photograph shows the floor of the left atrium looked at from above, with the mitral valve leaflets in the base. Note the ballooning of the mitral valve leaflets.

Q132. What is this condition called?

Q133. What is the underlying structural abnormality in the valve leaflets?

Q134. What are the clinical consequences?

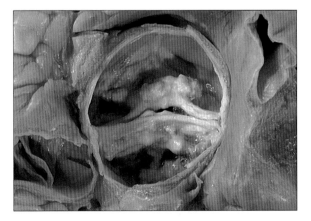

This is a photograph of the aortic valve seen from above.

Q135. Describe the abnormality of the valve.

Q136. What is the most likely diagnosis?

Q137. What other disease can produce this type of change in the aortic valve?

Q138. What are the haemodynamic consequences?

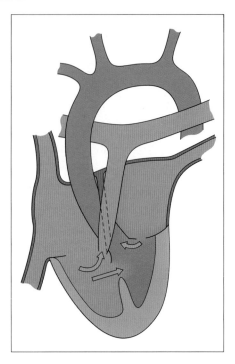

This diagram illustrates the features of the important congenital heart disease of children known as **Fallot's tetralogy**.

Q139. What are the four features of this tetralogy?

Q140. What are the haemodynamic consequences of this malformation?

Q141. What are the aims in surgical correction?

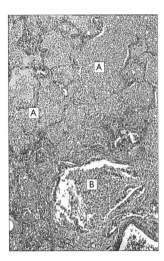

This histological section shows the lung histology of a 78-year-old man who developed fever and rapid respiratory rate, with râles and rhonci, for 2 days before his death. He had been admitted in deep coma with a dense left hemiplegia 5 days before his death.

Q142. What are the structures labelled **A** and **B**?

Q143. What is the purplish-staining material they contain?

Q144. What is the diagnosis, and how has the disease come to affect the lung?

Q145. What factors have predisposed to the disease in this man?

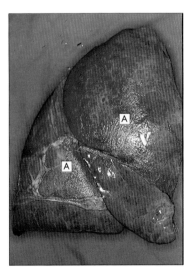

This lung was removed at post-mortem examination from a 43-year-old vagrant who was admitted moribund. His drinking friends said that he had been complaining of pain in the right side of his chest and had a cough which made the pain worse.

Q146. What is the cause of his chest pain?

Q147. What is the underlying lung disease?

Q148. What is the material labelled **A** adherent to the pleural surface?

Q149. What physical signs would be noted on listening to the right side of the chest with a stethoscope?

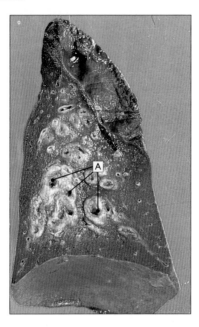

Q150. What are the structures labelled **A** in this photograph of a slice through the lobe of a lung?
Q151. What is the name of the disease?
Q152. What are the two main factors in the development of this condition?
Q153. Name four complications.

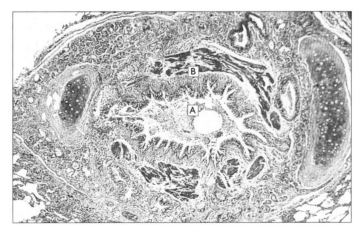

This photomicrograph shows a large branch bronchus from a patient with chronic asthma.

Q154. What is the material labelled **A** almost obliterating the bronchial lumen?

Q155. What is the feature of chronic asthma labelled **B**?

Q156. What type of immunological disorder plays a rôle in most cases of asthma?

Q157. What is the combination of asthma, chronic bronchitis and emphysema commonly called?

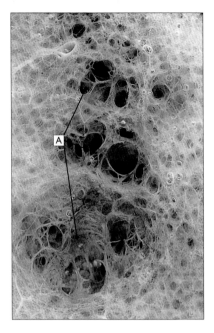

This photograph of the surface of the lung shows dilated air spaces (**A**) in **centriacinar emphysema.**

Q158. What is the other pattern of generalised emphysema?

Q159. What are the air spaces which are permanently distended in centriacinar emphysema?

Q160. What are the air spaces distended in the other pattern of generalised emphysema?

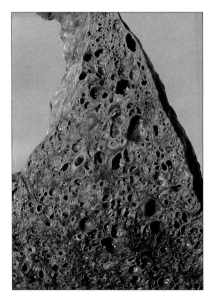

This photograph shows the cut surface of the lung of a patient who was known to have scleroderma with severe skin, renal and pulmonary involvement. She had developed progressively severe breathlessness over many years and a diagnosis of chronic interstitial fibrosis had been made.

Q161. What is this appearance called?

Q162. What are the main histological features?

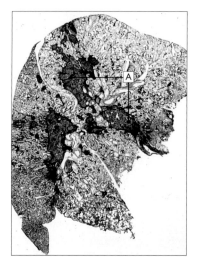

This thin slice through the lung shows the features of progressive massive fibrosis in a man with a long history of chest trouble.

Q163. What is the composition of the areas labelled **A**?

Q164. Why are they black?

Q165. What is the patient's previous occupation?

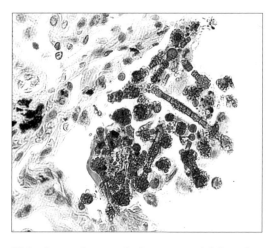

This photomicrograph shows material found histologically in the lung of a man who died of progressive chronic pulmonary fibrosis. He had worked in a shipyard for many years as a 'lagger'.

Q166. What is the brown material, and how did it gain access to the lungs?

Q167. What other lung disorders are associated with this material?

Q168. Is his former occupation significant?

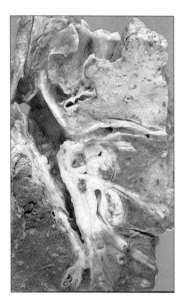

This photograph shows the lung removed at post-mortem from a man with a history of progressive breathlessness, recurrent lower lobe chest infections and haemoptysis. Chest radiograph showed a mass at the right lung hilum.

Q169. What is the abnormality?
Q170. What is the most likely histological appearance?
Q171. Why did the patient have haemoptysis?
Q172. Why did the patient have recurrent chest infections?

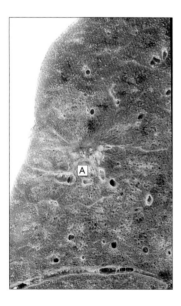

This photograph shows the cut surface of the lung with a peripheral irregular nodule (**A**). The patient had numerous intracerebral and intrahepatic tumour deposits.

Q173. What is the likely diagnosis?
Q174. What is the likely histological appearance?
Q175. What factors predispose to the development of this disorder?
Q176. What is the relationship between the lung, brain and liver changes?

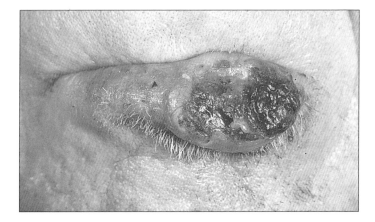

Q177. What is this large ulcerating lesion on the lip of an elderly man?

Q178. What are its main patterns of spread?

Q179. Where else in the mouth may this condition arise?

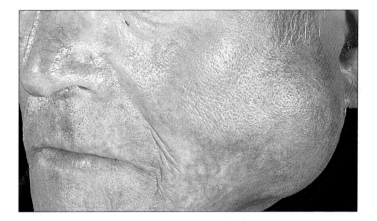

This elderly man has a large swelling at the angle of the jaw in front of the ear that has been slowly enlarging over many years.

Q180. Which organ or tissue is abnormal?

Q181. What is the most likely diagnosis?

Q182. What is the main hazard associated with surgical treatment?

Q183. What are the other possibilities in the differential diagnosis?

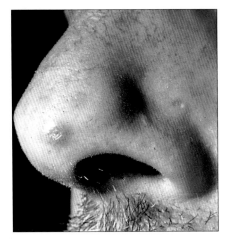

Q184. What is this lesion on the nose of an elderly man?

Q185. Is its appearance typical?

Q186. What is the behaviour of this lesion?

Q187. What aetiological factor is most important in the origin of this lesion?

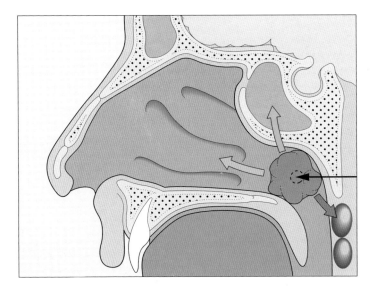

This artwork demonstrates the main clinical manifestations and complications of carcinoma of the nasopharynx. The yellow arrow indicates nasal obstruction and nose bleeds, while the blue arrow indicates local invasion of the VIth cranial nerve, leading to diplopia.

Q188. The red arrow indicates a common presenting feature of this tumour. What is it?

Q189. The pointer to the centre of the brown area indicates that the tumour may block the lower end of the Eustachian tube. What are the consequences of this?

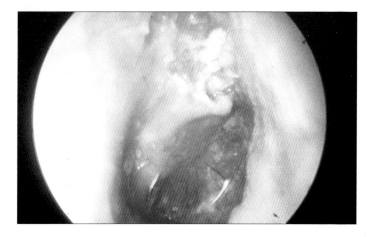

This photograph is an auroscopic view of the eardrum in a patient who has had an eardrum perforation in the attic region (top left).

Q190. What is the irregular white mass protruding through the area of the old perforation?

Q191. What is its histological appearance?

Q192. What are the complications of this lesion?

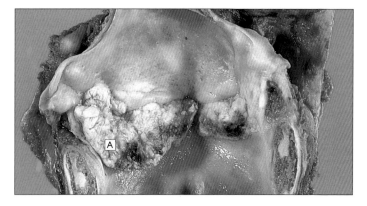

This photograph shows a total laryngectomy specimen dissected after fixation to show the larynx.

Q193. What is the structure labelled **A**?

Q194. What is the most likely presenting symptom?

Q195. How are these lesions classified by location, and what are the prognostic implications?

Q196. How do these lesions spread?

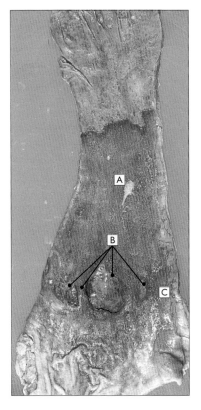

This photograph shows the lower oesophagus and upper stomach from a patient with a long history of gastro-oesophageal reflux, and shows the features of Barrett's oesophagus.

Q197. What do the labels **A**, **B** and **C** signify?

Q198. What is the mechanism leading to Barrett's oesophagus?

Q199. What are the complications of Barrett's oesophagus?

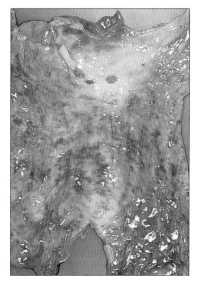

This opened stomach was removed at post-mortem from a man aged 48 who was admitted because of severe haematemesis and died before blood transfusion could be commenced. He had suffered from ankylosing spondylitis for many years, and was also a heavy drinker.

Q200. What abnormality does the gastric mucosa show?

Q201. What are the conditions which can produce this change?

Q202. What are the most likely causes in this man?

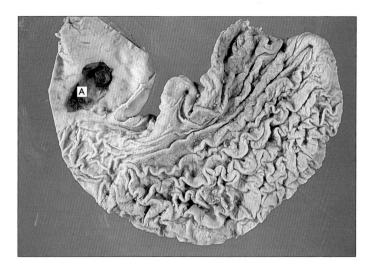

Q203. What is the lesion labelled **A** in the pyloric region of the stomach?

Q204. What factors predispose to this change in the stomach?

Q205. What are the most important complications?

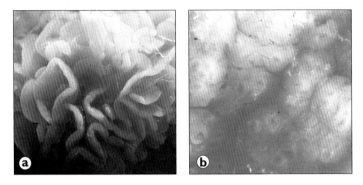

These two photographs show the dissecting microscopic appearances of jejunal mucosa; one is from a normal child; the other is from an underweight child who was failing to thrive.
Q206. Which is which?
Q207. What are the characteristic features seen here of the abnormal jejunal mucosa?
Q208. What is the most likely disease?
Q209. What is its pathogenesis?

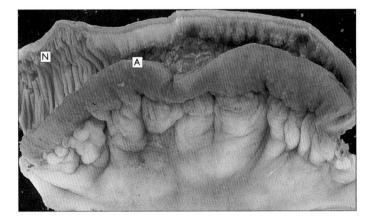

This segment of small bowel was removed at emergency laparotomy from a 32-year-old woman with subacute small bowel obstruction.
Q210. The area labelled **N** is normal. What is wrong at **A**, the site of subacute obstruction?
Q211. What is the most likely diagnosis?
Q212. Where else may this disease occur?
Q213. What are the main direct complications?

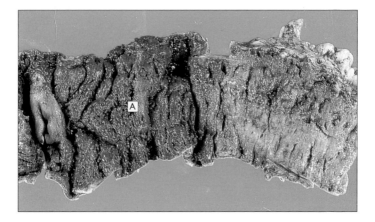

This photograph shows the mucosal appearances of a total colectomy specimen removed from a 32-year-old woman with a 5-year-history of intermittent severe diarrhoea, which is not responding to treatment.

Q214. What is the diagnosis?

Q215. How does the pattern of ulceration (**A**) differ from that seen in Crohn's disease?

Q216. What are the three main patterns of disease behaviour?

Q217. What are the most important indications for total colectomy?

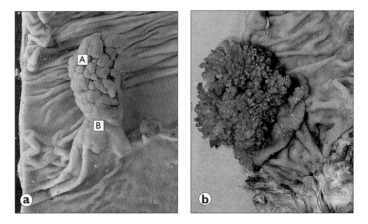

Photographs (a) and (b) show the two most important benign epithelial tumours of the large bowel.

Q218. What are they?

Q219. What is the difference between the two?

Q220. What are the most important complications?

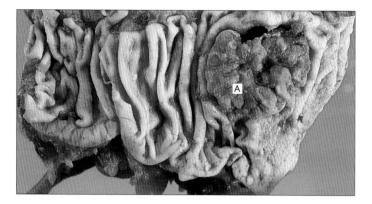

This photograph shows the descending colon and part of the rectum removed at operation.

Q221. What is the lesion labelled **A**?

Q222. How do such lesions present clinically?

Q223. What are the most important methods of spread?

Q224. What are the most prognostic features?

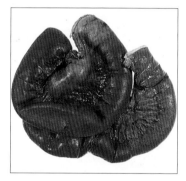

This loop of small bowel showed purplish/black discoloration when removed at postmortem examination from a man with a long history of ischaemic heart disease.

Q225. What is the diagnosis?

Q226. What are the three main causes?

Q227. Which is most likely in this patient?

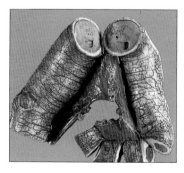

This photograph shows small bowel of an infant with meconium ileus in which the affected bowel is dilated and distended with thick green mucoid material.

Q228. What important genetic disease is meconium ileus an important manifestation of?

Q229. What are the pancreatic and pulmonary complications of that genetic disease?

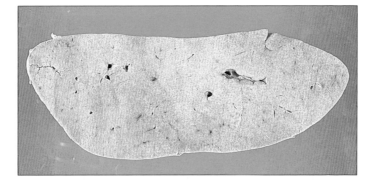

This photograph shows a slice of a large soft yellow liver removed at post-mortem from a 48-year-old man who was found dead in the basement of a derelict house surrounded by empty bottles of cheap wine.

Q230. What is the yellow colour due to?

Q231. What is the likely histological appearance?

Q232. What is the most likely cause in this case?

Q233. What other diseases can produce a soft yellow liver?

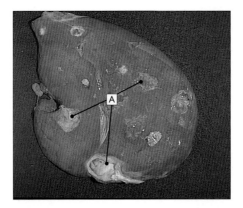

Q234. What are the lesions labelled **A** in this liver?

Q235. What are the three main routes used by bacteria to gain access to the liver?

Q236. What non-invasive techniques can be used to image these lesions in life?

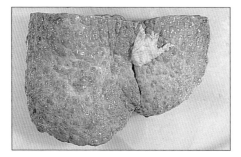

This photograph shows the liver from a woman aged 53 who died of liver failure after a long illness. Her terminal episode was a massive haematemesis.

Q237. What is the cause of the irregular appearance of the liver surface?

Q238. What are the three key histological features of this disease?

Q239. What is the likely cause of her massive haematemesis and what is the mechanism?

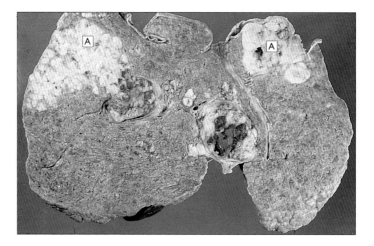

This photograph shows a slice through a liver from a 64-year-old man with a long history of cirrhosis of the liver, presumed to be alcoholic in origin.

Q240. What are the areas labelled **A**?

Q241. What are the factors which predispose to the development of the lesions **A**?

Q242. What serum tumour marker may be used to aid diagnosis in life?

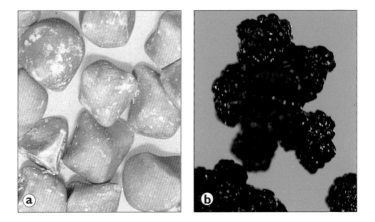

Photographs (a) and (b) show two types of gallstones removed from the gallbladders of two different people at cholecystectomy.

Q243. What type of stone is shown in (a) and how do they form?

Q244. What type of stone is shown in (b) and how do they form?

Q245. What changes may be seen in the gallbladder that contains gallstones?

Q246. Is there an increased risk of gallbladder malignancy in patients with gallstones?

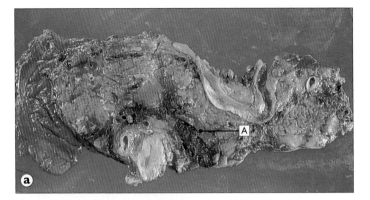

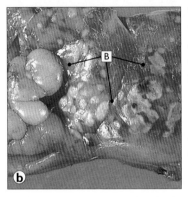

These photographs show (a) the cut surface appearance and (b) the surface appearance of the pancreas from a man aged 43 who was admitted as an emergency with abdominal pain and shock, dying shortly after arrival. He was a heavy 'social' drinker. The pancreas was soft, with extensive haemorrhagic areas (**A**) within it.

Q247. What is the most likely diagnosis?

Q248. What are the numerous small creamy/white patches labelled **B** in (b). How are they produced?

Q249. What blood enzyme level would have been useful in establishing the diagnosis in life?

Q250. What is the probable predisposing factor to the development of the disease in this case?

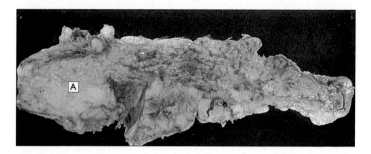

This is a pancreas removed at post-mortem from a 66-year-old man.

Q251. What is the lesion in the head of the pancreas indicated by the label (**A**)?

Q252. How does this disease tend to present clinically?

Q253. What prognosis does the disease carry?

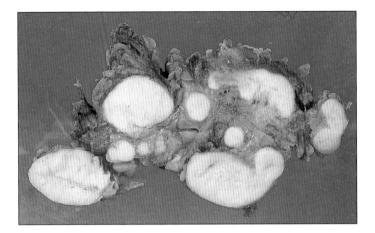

This photograph was taken from the neck region at post-mortem. The patient had masses in the neck, axillae and inguinal regions.

Q254. What are the well-circumscribed creamy white masses?

Q255. What are the possible diagnoses?

Q256. What is the most likely diagnosis?

Q257. How may an accurate diagnosis be established?

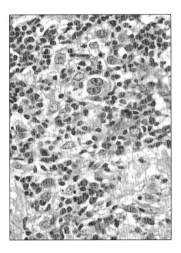

This photomicrograph shows the histological appearances of a lymph node from the patient with the enlarged cervical lymph nodes shown in **Q254–257**. One obvious feature is a large binucleate giant cell with two very similar nuclei, each with a prominent nucleolus.

Q258. What is the name given to this cell?

Q259. Which primary malignant lymphoma are these cells characteristic of?

Q260. How is this type of primary malignant lymphoma further classified?

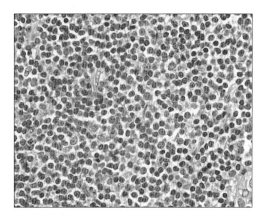

This photomicrograph shows the histological appearance of an enlarged lymph node from a 68-year-old man with generalised lymph node enlargement and anaemia. The normal lymph node architecture is destroyed and replaced by sheets of small lymphocytes with uniform nuclei and little cytoplasm.

Q261. What is the most likely diagnosis?

Q262. What is the most likely cause of his anaemia?

Q263. Why might this patient be predisposed to recurrent infections?

Q264. What is the prognosis in this type of disease?

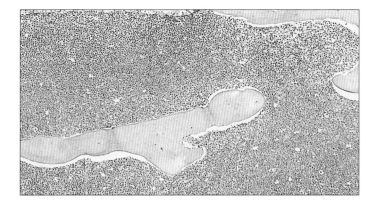

This photomicrograph shows the bone marrow from a patient who presented with severe anaemia and thrombocytopenia. The blood film showed abnormal circulating white cells.

Q265. How is the bone marrow abnormal in this photograph?

Q266. What is the most likely diagnosis?

Q267. How may an accurate diagnosis be obtained?

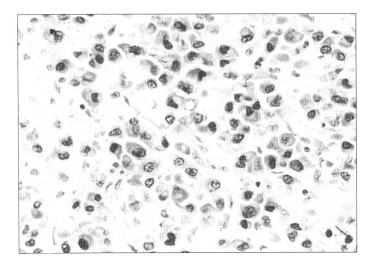

This photomicrograph shows the cells occupying much of the bone marrow cavity at an osteolytic lesion detected on X-ray in the right iliac crest. The patient presented with general bone pain and was found to have a leukoerythroblastic anaemia and proteinuria. Imaging had shown multiple osteolytic lesions in vertebrae, ribs, pelvic bones and skull.

Q268. What are these abnormal cells in the osteolytic lesions?
Q269. What is the diagnosis?
Q270. Why does the patient have leukoerythroblastic anaemia?
Q271. What are the possible causes for his proteinuria?

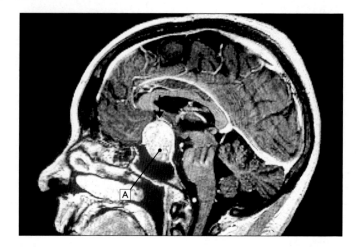

A 30-year-old man presents with progressive bitemporal hemianopia. This is the CT sagittal section of his head.

Q272. What abnormality is labelled **A**?

Q273. What is the cause of his visual disorder?

Q274. What other symptoms may the lesion shown in **A** manifest?

Q275. Which biblical character is thought to have had this lesion?

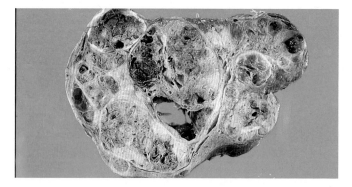

This photograph shows a slice of thyroid gland from a 66-year-old woman who had a subtotal thyroidectomy because of an unsightly swelling in her neck, present for many years.

Q276. What is the name of this disorder?

Q277. What is the brown material in some of the spaces, and why is it brown?

Q278. This lesion was removed for cosmetic reasons. What are the other indications for surgical removal?

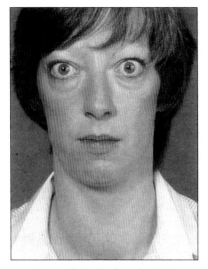

This clinical photograph shows the characteristic appearance of a patient with an important thyroid disorder.

Q279. What is the thyroid disorder?

Q280. What functional thyroid abnormality is associated with this disease?

Q281. What is the cause of the thyroid functional abnormality?

Q282. What is the name given to the characteristic eye appearances?

From C.D. Forbes & W.F. Jackson, *A Colour Atlas and Text of Clinical Medicine*, Mosby–Wolfe, London, 1993.

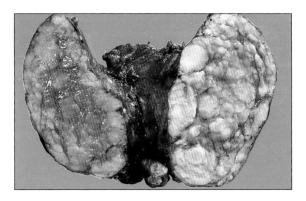

This photograph shows the cut surface of a symmetrically enlarged firm rubbery thyroid removed from the neck of a 43-year-old woman. The cut surface appearances are characteristic.

Q283. What is the disease?

Q284. Why is the cut surface white instead of brown?

Q285. What laboratory test may be used to diagnose this condition?

Q286. What is the impact of this disease on thyroid function?

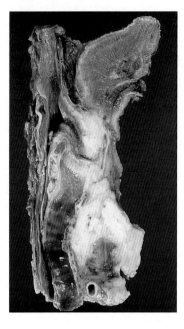

This photograph shows a section through the tongue, trachea and larynx of a woman aged 78 who presented with stridor and a rapidly enlarging lump in her neck.

Q287. Why did she have stridor?

Q288. What is the lump in the neck (seen in the photograph as irregular white tissue anterior to the trachea) most likely to have been?

Q289. What is the characteristic age incidence and behaviour of this disease?

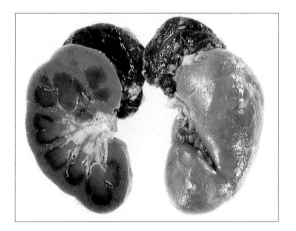

This photograph shows the kidneys and adrenals from a child who died suddenly after a brief history of an acute feverish illness with lethargy.

Q290. What abnormality do the adrenals show?

Q291. What is the name of this syndrome?

Q292. What is the most likely cause of this child's fatal feverish illness?

Q293. What are the cutaneous manifestations of this disease?

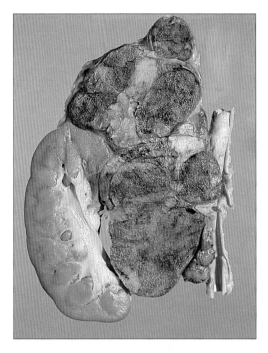

This photograph shows the right kidney and part of a large abdominal mass in a child aged 3 who died of widespread malignancy.

Q294. What is the malignant tumour and what is its tissue of origin?

Q295. What are the most likely sites for metastatic spread of this tumour?

Q296. What laboratory tests may be used to establish the diagnosis in life?

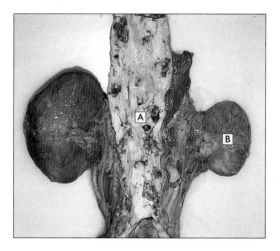

This photograph shows the kidneys removed at post-mortem from a 68-year-old woman who died of a massive cerebral haemorrhage originating in the basal ganglia region on the right.

Q297. What is the structure labelled **A** and what disease does it show?

Q298. Why do you think the kidney labelled **B** is smaller than normal, and the kidney on the other side larger than normal?

Q299. What is the relationship between these abnormalities and the mode of death?

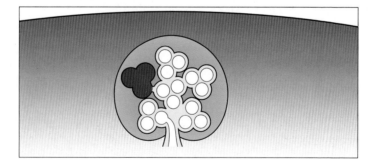

This drawing is a diagrammatic representation of a glomerulus in the cortex of the kidney. The majority of the glomerulus (white) is normal, but there is one part of the glomerular capillary system which is diseased (red).

Q300. What is the name given to this pattern of glomerular abnormality?

Q301. What do the terms 'global', 'diffuse' and 'focal' mean when applied to glomerular disease?

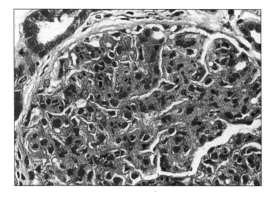

This photomicrograph shows part of a glomerulus from a renal biopsy sample taken from a 7-year-old boy who presented with a 2-week history of passing only small amounts of dark brown urine, general malaise and some swelling of the face, particularly around the eyes. A urine sample showed the presence of blood (haematuria) and he was noted to be hypertensive, with a raised blood urea and blood creatinine. He had complained of a sore throat approximately 10 days before the onset of this illness.

Q302. What syndrome does this child have?

Q303. In the photomicrograph most of the glomerular capillary lumina are occluded. What is responsible?

Q304. What is the name given to this glomerular disease?

Q305. What is the likely outcome in this case?

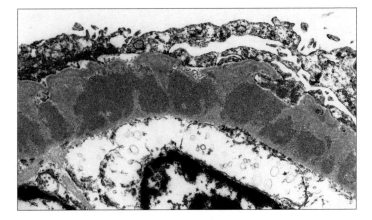

This electron micrograph shows the glomerular capillary basement membrane from a 75-year-old man with a 2-month history of progressive lethargy and pallor associated with puffy swelling of the fingers, hands and feet. He reported that his urine seemed thick and very frothy. Laboratory investigations showed severe proteinuria, and he had a very low serum albumin. The electron micrograph shows electron-dense immune complexes incorporated into a thickened glomerular basement membrane.

Q306. What is the name given to the clinical syndrome with which this patient presented?

Q307. What are the key features of the syndrome and how are they interrelated?

Q308. The changes shown in this electron micrograph were uniform throughout all glomeruli examined (global and diffuse). By light microscopy, all glomerular basement membranes were noted to be thickened. What is the name given to the glomerular disease demonstrated by this electron micrograph?

Q309. What is a likely precipitating factor for this disease in a patient of this age?

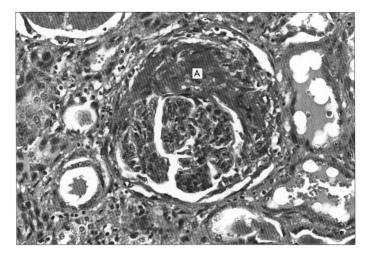

This photomicrograph shows a glomerulus from a renal biopsy from a man aged 58 with renal failure of rapid progression. He presented with malaise persisting after a viral illness, developed puffiness of the face, hands and feet and noticed brown discoloration of the urine. His urine output had progressively fallen over the 10 days prior to admission, and at the time of the biopsy he was passing no urine (anuria). Investigations showed a high blood urea and creatinine, with blood in the few drops of urine he was passing each day.

Q310. What is the lesion labelled **A** and what is its impact on the glomerulus and its function?

Q311. What is this type of glomerular disease called?

Q312. Renal biopsy showed that 17 out of the 19 glomeruli present showed lesions similar to **A**. What is the prognosis?

Q313. What is the likely cause in this case?

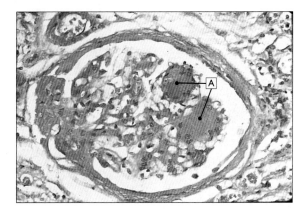

This photomicrograph shows a glomerulus taken from post-mortem kidney of a man aged 58 with a long history of medical disease which included progressive blindness and severe peripheral vascular disease necessitating bilateral amputation of his legs.

Q314. What are the homogeneous rounded lesions (**A**) in the glomerular tuft?

Q315. What are they composed of?

Q316. Which general medical disease did this patient suffer from?

Q317. In what other ways does this disease affect the kidney?

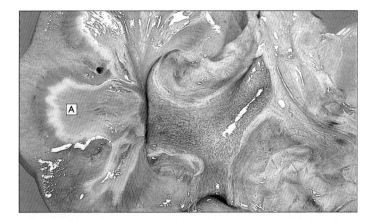

This photograph shows the cut surface of a kidney removed at post-mortem examination.

Q318. What is wrong with the area labelled **A**?

Q319. What are the important causes of this change?

Q320. What is the outcome of this abnormality?

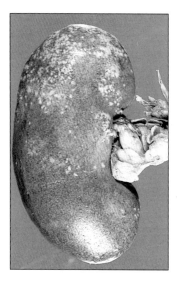

The photograph shows a kidney removed at autopsy from a 28-year-old woman who presented with rigors, a fever of 39.9°C, a pulse rate of 160 beats per minute, and a falling blood pressure of 80/40.

Q321. What clinical syndrome was developing when she presented?

Q322. What are the small white dots on the subcapsular surface of the kidney and how are they related to her clinical presentation?

Q323. How is the kidney likely to have developed this disease?

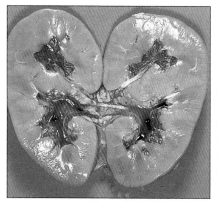

This photograph shows the cut surfaces of a kidney removed at autopsy from a young man who had been involved in a road traffic accident, sustaining severe internal injuries, including limb and pelvic fractures, lacerations to the liver and a ruptured spleen.

Emergency surgery, lasting 6 hours, was performed and he required substantial blood transfusion although his blood pressure remained low. The bleeding from the pelvic fractures was particularly difficult to control. After the operation he passed no urine and died 24 hours later despite full supportive measures. At post-mortem examination both kidneys showed this appearance of marked swelling and cortical pallor.

Q324. What is the diagnosis?

Q325. What would be seen histologically?

Q326. What are the possible causes of this lesion in this case?

Q327. What other disorders may produce this change?

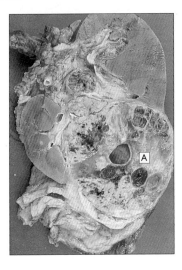

This kidney was removed at nephrectomy performed on a woman aged 50 who had painless haematuria and a palpable mass in the right loin.

Q328. What is the lesion labelled **A** and what is its cell or origin?

Q329. What is the natural history of this lesion?

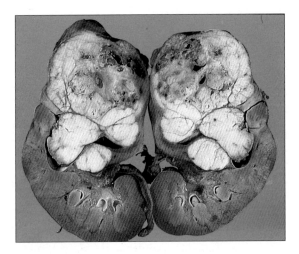

This photograph shows a kidney removed surgically from a 2-year-old child who presented with a large mass in the left loin and abdomen noticed by the mother.

Q330. What is the diagnosis?

Q331. Why?

Q332. What is the behaviour and prognosis?

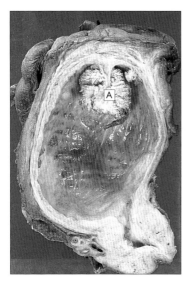

This photograph shows a bladder and prostate sectioned to show a lesion (**A**) at the fundus of the bladder.

Q333. What is the lesion labelled **A**? Is it benign or malignant?

Q334. Alongside it is a very similar but much smaller lesion. What is it?

Q335. How are these lesions graded?

Q336. What would have been this man's presenting symptom?

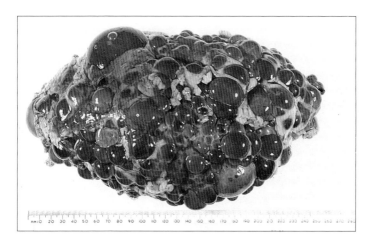

This photograph shows one of an identical pair of kidneys removed at post-mortem from a patient who died in a road traffic accident at the age of 43. He had never sought medical attention and was apparently well.

Q337. What is the disease?

Q338. What would have been found if this man had ever sought medical attention?

Q339. What is the more usual natural history of this disease?

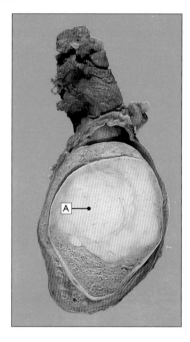

This photomicrograph shows an orchidectomy specimen from a man aged 42 who presented with painless swelling of the testis.

Q340. What is the lesion labelled **A** within the testis?

Q341. What is the evidence for your diagnosis?

Q342. What is the behaviour of this lesion?

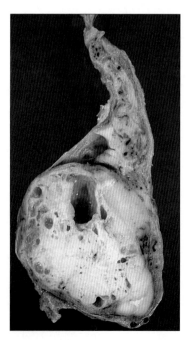

This photograph shows a transected testis removed at orchidectomy from a man aged 28 with a unilateral painless testicular swelling.

Q343. What is the diagnosis?

Q344. What is the evidence for your diagnosis?

Q345. What is the behaviour of this disorder?

Q346. What is the value of tumour cell markers in this disease?

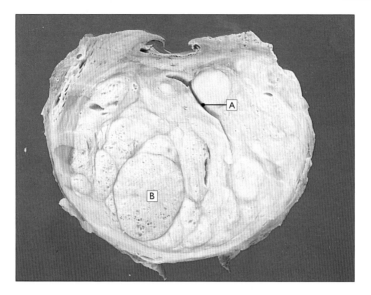

This photograph shows a section through the prostate gland of a man aged 74.

Q347. What does the shape of structure **A** indicate, and how might this be related to his likely presenting symptoms?

Q348. What is the disease, and what does the label **B** indicate?

Q349. How would you examine this organ clinically, and what would you expect to find?

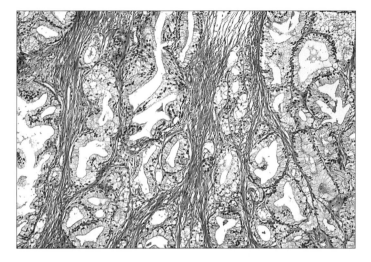

This photomicrograph, showing irregular distorted glandular structures, was prepared from a needle biopsy of the prostate gland. The patient was a man of 58 who was being investigated for severe lower back pain; radiography of the lumbar spine showed rounded areas of increased bone density in L4 and L5. The surgeon performed a rectal examination and found a hard irregular craggy enlargement of the prostate.

Q350. What is the diagnosis?

Q351. Why did the radiological appearances point to the prostate?

Q352. How was the needle biopsy obtained?

Q353. What is the behaviour of this tumour, and what is the value of tumour markers?

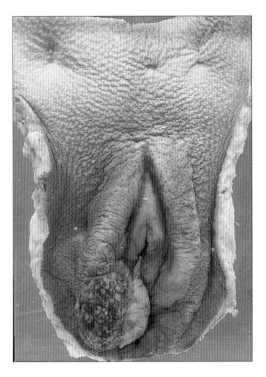

This photograph shows a radical vulvectomy specimen.
Q354. What is the abnormality?
Q355. What is its behaviour?
Q356. What is the usual age incidence?
Q357. Which lymph nodes drain this region?

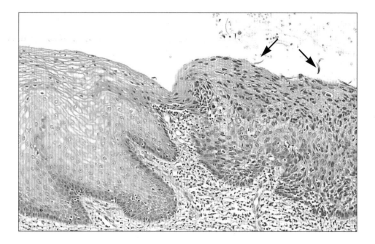

This photomicrograph was taken from a biopsy of the uterine cervix of a woman aged 40. It shows two different patterns of epithelium—one normal, the other abnormal.

Q358. Which side is normal and which is abnormal?

Q359. What are the important features of the abnormal epithelium?

Q360. What is the name given to this condition and how may it be diagnosed?

Q361. What are the risks of this epithelial abnormality?

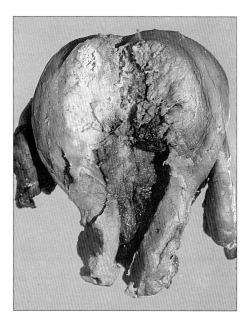

The photograph shows the uterus from a 68-year-old woman who presented with post-menopausal bleeding.

Q362. What is the diagnosis?

Q363. How is the diagnosis established clinically?

Q364. What is the behaviour of this disease?

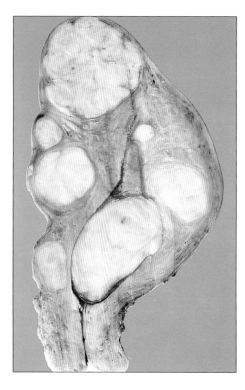

This photograph shows a section through a uterus removed from a woman aged 39 who complained of heavy irregular and painful periods.

Q365. What are the well-circumscribed white lesions in the uterus?

Q366. Why do they cause heavy periods?

Q367. What is the natural history of lesions if there is no surgical intervention?

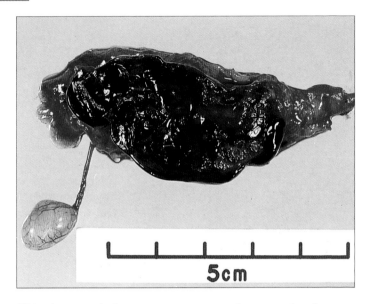

This photograph shows an organ removed at operation from a young woman aged 23 who was admitted as an emergency, having collapsed while shopping in a supermarket. When admitted to the Accident and Emergency Department, she had severe abdominal pain in the right iliac fossa, with tenderness and guarding, a pulse of 160 beats per minute, and a blood pressure of 100/50.

Q368. What is the organ?

Q369. What is the abnormality?

Q370. Why are her vital signs abnormal in the Accident and Emergency Department?

Q371. What factors predispose to this condition?

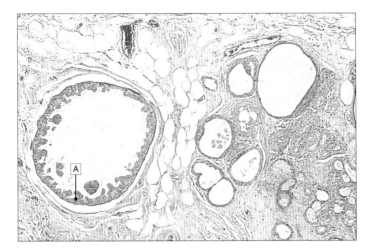

The photomicrograph shows a section from an excision biopsy of an irregular rubbery lump in the left breast of a 29-year-old woman. The lump had been present for some weeks and the patient's attention had been drawn to it because it was tender just before her period. She felt the lump tended to vary in size, being bigger just before menstruation.

Q372. What breast disease is demonstrated here?

Q373. What does the label **A** indicate?

Q374. What are the main pathological features of the disease?

Q375. What percentage of women have clinical symptoms of this disease?

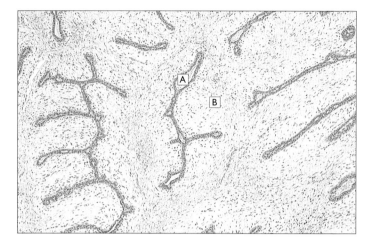

This photomicrograph shows part of a well-circumscribed 2-cm diameter solitary lump removed from the upper outer quadrant of the right breast in a 23-year-old woman.

Q376. What is this lesion and what do labels **A** and **B** indicate?
Q377. Is this condition benign or malignant?

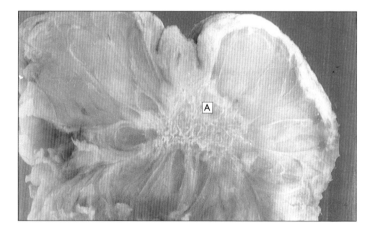

This photograph shows a slice through the breast removed at mastectomy from a 53-year-old woman complaining of a hard irregular lump immediately beneath the nipple, which had become retracted.

Q378. What is the lesion labelled **A**?
Q379. Why has the nipple become retracted?
Q380. Why are these lesions frequently hard and craggy on palpation?
Q381. What is the behaviour of these lesions?

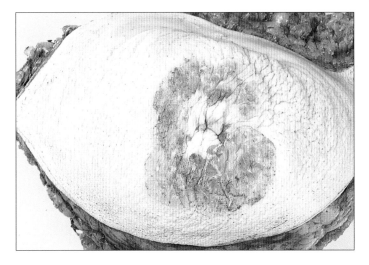

This photograph shows a mastectomy specimen from a woman of 69 who had an expanding irregular red thickening of the skin of the breast, centred on the nipple. It had started as a scaly red patch on the nipple; the patient had thought it was dermatitis and had been treating the area with a proprietary cream. She eventually sought medical advice when the lesion had reached the extent shown, and central ulceration had largely destroyed the nipple.

Q382. What was the original red skin 'rash'?

Q383. Why did she require mastectomy?

Q384. What is the basis of the skin changes in the nipple in this condition?

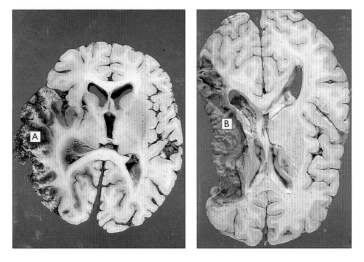

The above brain slices were both taken from patients who died with dense hemiplegia as a result of a stroke.

Q385. What are the lesions labelled **A** and **B**?

Q386. One patient died in deep coma within a couple of days of developing the hemiplegia, the other survived, hemiplegic, eventually dying of a myocardial infarct 2 years later. Which is which?

Q387. In which vascular territory have the abnormalities arisen?

Q388. What are the most likely causes of the lesions shown?

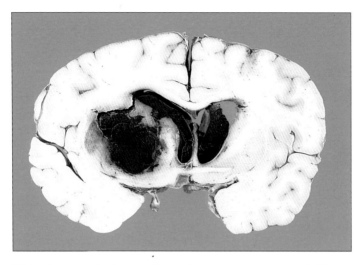

This photograph shows a slice of brain from a man aged 63 who collapsed and died suddenly.

Q389. What is the abnormality?

Q390. Where is it located?

Q391. What other systemic disease is the patient highly likely to have?

Q392. Why is this area of the brain the most common site for this disorder?

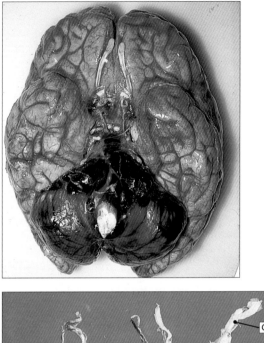

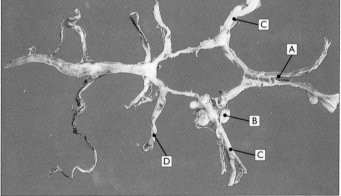

The brain was removed at post-mortem from a 33-year-old man who collapsed and died while playing golf. He began to complain of a headache on the 4th tee, and by the time he reached the green (in 5!) he felt he could not carry on because of rapid worsening of his headache. His playing partner escorted him back to the Club House, but he collapsed and died in the changing room.

Q393. What abnormality does the brain show?

Q394. What is its association with the other photograph shown here?

Q395. How may this condition be diagnosed in life?

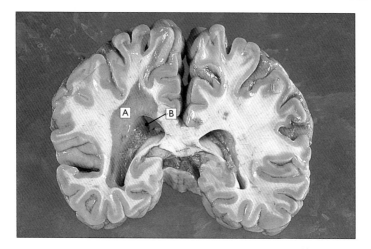

This photograph shows a slice of brain removed at post-mortem from a woman aged 47 with a long history of an intermittently progressive neurological disease.

Q396. The label **B** identifies a lateral ventricle. What is the lesion **A**?

Q397. What progressive neurological disorder did she suffer from?

Q398. There were similar smaller lesions scattered throughout the white matter of the cerebrum, cerebellum and brain stem. Is this typical?

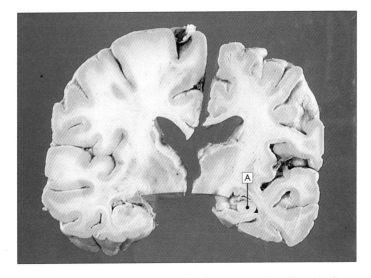

This photograph shows slices of half of the cerebral hemisphere from two patients: left, from a healthy 70-year-old man; right, from a patient of the same age who had been under care because of progressive dementia.

Q399. What are the features of the brain from the patient with dementia?

Q400. What is the region identified as **A** and why is it important in dementias?

Q401. What is the most likely cause of this patient's dementia?

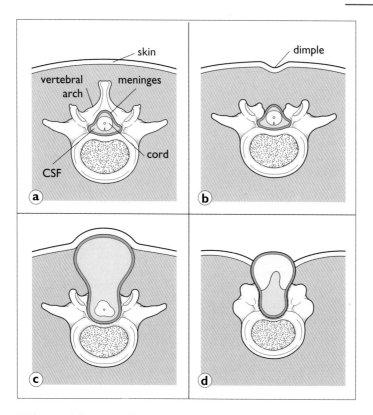

This set of diagrams shows the varying degrees of the clinically important neural tube defects which are most common in the lumbar region. Drawing (a) indicates the normal structure.

Q402. What is the name given to the lesion in (b) and what is the abnormality?

Q403. What is the name given to the lesion in (c) and what is the abnormality?

Q404. What is the name given to the lesion in (d) and what is the abnormality?

Q405. What clinical features are associated with (c) and (d), including intracranial lesions?

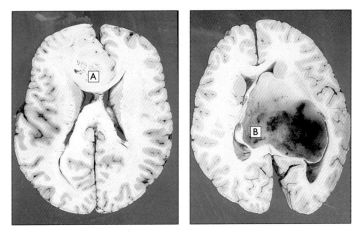

These two photographs of brain slices each show gliomas, labelled **A** and **B**, respectively: one is well-differentiated, with no histological atypia and a slow rate of growth, while the other is a highly malignant glial tumour with a rapid rate of growth.

Q406. Which is which?

Q407. What enables you to distinguish the two types with the naked eye?

Q408. What is the prognosis in the two types illustrated?

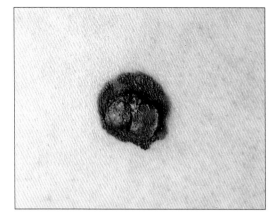

This photograph shows a lesion from the thigh of a 27-year-old woman. It had started as a flat pigmented patch, but had developed a raised central nodule in the 2 weeks before admission.

Q409. What is the diagnosis?

Q410. What was the early flat lesion in which the raised nodular lesion developed?

Q411. Is this a good prognosis or poor prognosis lesion?

Q412. If spread were to occur, what is the first likely site?

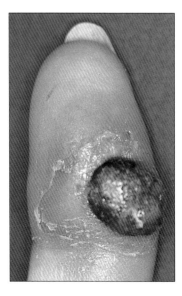

This photograph shows a frightening-looking skin lesion commonly seen in family and clinic/office practice. Such lesions grow rapidly to produce pedunculated red nodules. The finger is a common site as are the head and neck and the gingival mucosa.

Q413. What is this lesion called?

Q414. What is a frequent precipitating factor on the finger?

Q415. Which particular group of people develop similar lesions on the gingival mucosa?

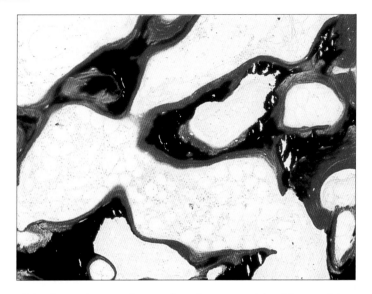

This photomicrograph was taken from a trephine biopsy of the bone of the iliac crest and has been stained to show the distinction between mineralised bone (black) and unmineralised osteoid (red). The patient was a 45-year-old woman who had lived in the UK for 20 years, having been born and brought up in Calcutta.

Q416. What is the name of the disease, and what are the characteristic histological features shown in the photomicrograph?

Q417. What is the pathogenesis of the disease?

Q418. What are the likely mechanisms in this particular patient?

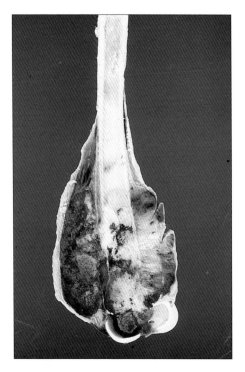

This photograph shows the femur from a boy aged 10.

Q419. What is the large mass at the lower end?

Q420. What is the behaviour of this disease?

Q421. Is the age and sex incidence and location typical?

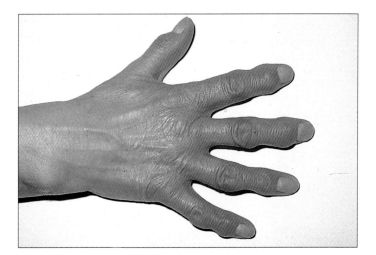

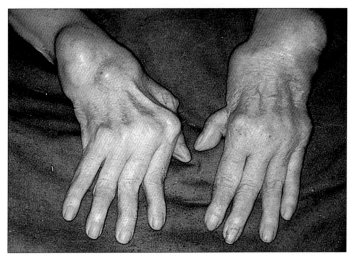

Both of these patients had a long history of painful swollen joints in the fingers, and the photographs show the two most common forms of joint disease, osteoarthritis and rheumatoid arthritis.
Q422. Which is which and why?
Q423. What is the basis of the disease in each case?

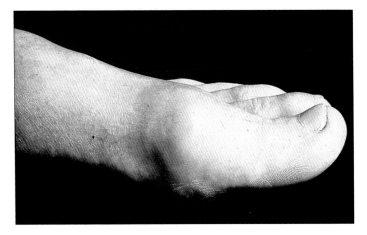

This photomicrograph shows the big toe of a man aged 47 with a history of recurrent attacks of acute pain and swelling in the joint shown.

Q424. What is the diagnosis?

Q425. How else may this disease manifest?

Q426. What local and systemic complications may occur?

A1. (b) shows skeletal muscle **hypertrophy.**
A2. The most likely stimulus to the adaptive change is increased work (e.g. sporting activity).
A3. (i) **hypertrophy;** (ii) **hyperplasia.**
See *Pathology*, p.13.

A4. The prostatic urethra.
A5. Hyperplasia (benign prostatic hyperplasia).
A6. A nodule of hyperplastic prostatic tissue composed of hyperplastic glands and stroma.
A7. Symptoms—poor urinary stream, difficulty starting micturition, terminal dribbling. Also frequency, nocturia and occasionally urgency.
Physical signs—smooth, usually symmetrical, nodular enlargement of prostate palpable on rectal examination. Texture is rubbery and firm, as opposed to craggy and hard (usually an indication of prostatic carcinoma).
Complications—chronic urinary retention with bladder hypertrophy and predisposition to ascending urinary infection and calculus formation. Risk of episodes of acute urinary retention. Long-term risk of chronic renal failure and papillary necrosis.
See *Pathology*, p.15.

A8. The adrenal in (a) is smaller than normal, mainly as a result of reduction in size of the pale yellowish white adrenal cortex, which has undergone symmetrical **atrophy.**
A9. The most likely cause is from the prolonged administration of corticosteroids used in the treatment of patients with severe rheumatoid arthritis. The therapeutic steroids interfere with the normal feedback mechanism, fooling the pituitary–adrenal axis into believing that the adrenal cortex is producing adequate or excessive hormone. The pituitary, therefore, puts out little or no ACTH and the adrenal cortex becomes structurally and functionally atrophic.
A10. If corticosteroid therapy is stopped abruptly, the patient may develop an acute adrenal crisis because the atrophic cortex is unable to replace the missing corticosteroids instantly. This is called an Addisonian crisis and can be rapidly fatal. In addition, prolonged corticosteroid therapy can produce the symptoms of Cushing's syndrome.
See *Pathology*, p.19.

A11. The vacuoles contain lipids; this is called 'fatty change'.
A12. Diabetes/starvation (increased mobilisation of free fatty acids).
  Alcohol (increased conversion of fatty acids to triglycerides).
  Hypoxia/toxins (reduced oxidation of triglycerides).
  Protein malnutrition (reduced lipid acceptor proteins).

A13. The most likely cause is **alcoholic liver disease**, the most important complication of which is **cirrhosis of the liver**.
See *Pathology*, p.28.

A14. (a) Cytoplasmic vacuolation.
(b) Pyknosis.
(c) Karyorrhexis.
(d) Karyolysis.

A15. Cytoplasmic vacuolation is the earliest indication of cell damage, and is potentially recoverable.

Pyknosis is characterised by the cell nuclei becoming small and densely stained (indicating cessation of DNA transcription), with shrunken and densely stained cytoplasm.

Karyorrhexis is fragmentation of the pyknotic nucleus into small pieces as a result of the autolytic activity of nucleases.

Karyolysis is the result of continuing nuclease breakdown, producing complete dissolution of the karyorrhexic nuclear fragments. The shrunken eosinophilic cytoplasm begins to fragment.

A16. The normal sequence is:
Cytoplasmic vacuolation→ pyknosis→ karyorrhexis→ karyolysis
See *Pathology*, p.29.

A17. Figure (a) shows coagulative necrosis, in which the architecture of the dead tissue is still recognisable.
Figure (b) shows colliquative necrosis in which no original structure can be determined, the tissue being replaced by fluid, necrotic debris, and phagocytic cells.

A18. The organ involved in coagulative necrosis is the kidney; **A** is the glomerulus and **B** the tubules; note that the architecture is identifiable although all cells are necrotic and devoid of nuclei.

A19. The organ most likely to be involved in colliquative necrosis is the brain, as in the photomicrograph above. Note that it is impossible to identify that this tissue is brain since the necrotic area shows no viable or ghost residue of normal structure.

A20. Both these types of necrosis are due to **infarction**.

A21. The area of coagulative necrosis will heal by organisation and fibrosis to form a small fibrous scar. The area of colliquative necrosis in the brain will result in a cystic lesion containing fluid and surrounded by dense gliosis produced by reactive astrocytes.
See *Pathology*, p.31.

A22. A = cardiac muscle; **B** = amylase.

A23. You need to measure the cardiac enzymes and serum amylase. With the patient's history as given, acute pancreatitis associated with an episode of recent heavy alcohol intake is the most likely diagnosis. Myocardial infarction is always a possibility, since it is not invariably associated with pain localisable to the chest. Some patients complain of 'indigestion' or 'heartburn'.

A24. The enzymes must be measured sequentially since they are released into the blood at different stages after myocardial fibre necrosis. Creatine kinase: MB reaches a peak approximately 24 hours after infarction and falls away rapidly between 36 and 48 hours. AST and LDH1 (or hydroxybutyrate dehydrogenase: HBD) are scarcely raised at 24 hours; they reach a peak between 1 and 3 days, before slowly falling away. The persistence of a raised creatine kinase for 2 or 3 days after the onset of chest pain suggests continuing extension of the infarct.
See *Pathology*, p.32.

A25. A = lymphatic spread by tumour eroding through lymphatic walls, and clumps of tumour cells breaking off and passing in the lymphatic channels.
B = spread by local invasion into adjacent tissue.
C = bloodstream or haematogenous spread by tumour eroding through thin-walled blood vessels (usually venules and veins), and tumour cells breaking off and passing into the blood circulation.
D = transcoelomic spread by tumour cells eroding through a mesothelial surface and passing into a coelomic space, with cells breaking off and passing in the space to other sites where they implant elsewhere on the surface. In this case, the coelomic space is the pleural cavity.
A26. Common sites for bloodstream spread of lung cancer are liver, bone, brain, and adrenals, but bloodstream spread may be extensive and involve many organs, particularly in small-celled undifferentiated carcinoma.
See *Pathology*, p.38.

A27. A = aorta (abdominal), **B** = inferior vena cava, **C** = para-aortic lymph nodes.
A28. A shows severe atherosclerosis, particularly in the section just above the bifurcation into iliac arteries.
A29. The para-aortic lymph nodes (**C**) are greatly enlarged by fleshy white tumour.
A30. The tumour in **C** may be a primary tumour of lymph nodes, such as a malignant lymphoma, or a metastatic tumour spread to the para-aortic lymph nodes via lymphatics from their primary site. The kidneys and pelvic organs drain into the para-aortic lymph nodes, so the primary tumour could be a malignant renal tumour, carcinomas of the endometrium, cervix or ovary or metastases from a malignant testicular tumour such as a seminoma. However, in the late stages the para-aortic lymph nodes may also be involved in tumours from other sites, such as the breast, bronchus or alimentary tract.
See *Pathology*, p.39.

A31. This is a strip of vertebral bodies from the lumbar vertebra, each bone block being separated from its neighbour by an intervertebral disc.

A32. The lesions labelled **A** are most likely to be deposits of metastatic malignant tumour, usually metastatic carcinoma.

A33. The tumours most likely to metastasise to bone are carcinomas of the **bronchus, breast, thyroid, kidney and prostate.** Among the many other malignant tumours which can metastasise to bone are neuroblastoma (in children) and testicular teratoma. Multiple tumour nodules in bone may also be due to **multiple myeloma**, although the tumour deposits are usually greyish red rather than white as here.

See *Pathology*, p. 40.

A34. The brain (a) shows a number of large tumour deposits, two of which are labelled **A**. The liver (b) shows large numbers of whitish tumour deposits of varying sizes, but all are spherical except where they are becoming confluent. The adrenal (c) is largely replaced by creamy white tumour deposit and only a thin rim of normal adrenal tissue can be seen stretched around the single tumour mass.

A35. In the same patient these are most likely to be metastatic tumour deposits spread via the bloodstream.

A36. In a patient of this age the most likely site of primary tumour is the lung, where the primary carcinoma is most likely to be found in the main bronchi near the hilum although quite small peripheral primary adenocarcinomas of the lung can produce large, extensive metastatic tumour deposits. In a man most cases of metastasis in the adrenals are from primary bronchial carcinomas.

A37. In most cases, metastases in the liver come from a primary in the alimentary tract via the portal venous system, although carcinoma of the breast is also a common primary site.

See *Pathology*, p. 40.

A38. Another common site in the alimentary tract is the colon, where progression through dysplasia to invasive carcinoma may occur in long-standing ulcerative colitis.

A39. Two other common sites for this sequence are the uterine cervix and the skin, where invasive carcinoma may be preceded by dysplasia and carcinoma *in situ.*

A40. Yes, invasive cancer may be prevented if the abnormal epithelium is completely excised or eradicated at the dysplasia/carcinoma in-situ stage.

A41. Histological examination of the abnormal epithelium removed by biopsy, or cytological examination of abnormal cells removed by exfoliation.

See *Pathology*, p. 44.

A42. A = **trophoblastic tumours** (such as trophoblastic tumours of the testis and choriocarcinoma of the endometrium), which produce excess HCG.
B = prostatic carcinomas, which produce **acid phosphatases.**
C = **endocrine tumours**, which produce hormone products.
A43. Tumour markers are assessed using blood samples.
A44. Monitoring of tumour markers may assist in the early diagnosis of residual or recurrent tumours. This is particularly important in trophoblastic tumours, where rising HCG levels after treatment indicate tumour recurrence.
See *Pathology*, p. 55.

A45. The vessel is persistently dilated, flow has slowed, and blood white cells are accumulating and adhering to the endothelial surface ('margination').
A46. The major cell type accumulating at this early stage is the neutrophil polymorph.
A47. In the next stage of the acute inflammatory reaction, neutrophils migrate through the blood vessel wall into the area of tissue damage, accompanied by fluid and fibrinogen from the vessel wall.
A48. The most common outcome is the formation of an acute inflammatory exudate, removal of necrotic debris and its replacement by vascular granulation tissue which then undergoes progressive fibrosis to form a collagenous scar at the site of tissue damage.
See *Pathology*, p. 60.

A49. The dark lines are prominent superficial blood vessels.
A50. The creamy material is an acute inflammatory exudate which is very rich in neutrophil polymorphs, making a thick cell-rich creamy exudate (purulent exudate).
A51. This is acute bacterial meningitis, and the most likely causative bacteria are *Haemophilus influenzae* and the meningococcus.
A52. It is important to establish that the patient has meningeal inflammation (i.e. some form of meningitis), that the inflammation is acute and bacterial, and to identify accurately the causative bacterium so that the correct antibiotic can be given. This is achieved by a combination of microscopic examination and microbiological culture of cerebrospinal fluid obtained by lumbar or cranial puncture.
See *Pathology*, p. 64.

A53. The pericardial surfaces show **acute fibrinous pericarditis,** an acute inflammatory reaction on both pericardial surfaces.
A54. In this case the exudate has a very high percentage of fibrin strands producing the thickened appearance seen, and neu-

trophils are a relatively minor component of the inflammatory exudate. This is a common feature where inflammation involves serosal surfaces: for example, pleura and peritoneum. In **Q49–52** the exudate has a high percentage of neutrophils and comparatively little fibrin, producing a creamy purulent fluid; purulent exudate is usually the result of bacterial infection.

A55. The most likely cause is damage to the pericardium resulting from **myocardial infarction**. Less common is viral or bacterial infection. The presence of a pericardial exudate may be manifest on examination by hearing a pericardial friction rub with every beat of the heart.

A56. The fibrinous exudate heals by granulation tissue formation and fibrous scarring producing fibrous pericardial adhesions which fuse the visceral to the parietal pericardium, with partial or complete obliteration of the pericardial cavity.
See *Pathology*, p. 64.

A57. Minimal disruption of supporting stroma and preservation of some epithelial cells to allow regeneration.

A58. When a damaging stimulus persists, complete healing cannot occur, and chronic inflammation occurs; the processes of continuing necrosis, organisation and repair all occur concurrently.

A59. Organisation of acute inflammatory exudate to form granulation tissue, which then undergoes fibrous replacement to form fibrous scar, is the most common outcome of tissue damage.
See *Pathology*, p. 68.

A60. The alveoli contain an acute inflammatory exudate largely composed of neutrophils mixed with some fibrin and fluid. This is pneumonic consolidation—in this particular case **lobar pneumonia**, because of the localisation of the consolidation to one lobe. The most likely cause is a bacterial infection, with the most likely causative organism being *Pneumococcus* or *Klebsiella*.

A61. The neutrophil-rich acute inflammatory exudate in the alveoli would have undergone **resolution**. Enzymes released by neutrophils break up the fibrin and any cell debris, and macrophages phagocytose any residual solid material before being reabsorbed into the lymphatic or blood vascular systems. The exudate is first rendered largely fluid and is then reabsorbed, permitting air to enter the alveolar spaces again. The alveolar sacs are re-lined with new epithelial cells and normal function returns. Resolution can occur only where there has been minimal structural damage; in lobar pneumonia the exudate forms in response to the presence of bacteria and their toxins, and structural damage is largely confined to destruction of alveolar lining cells. In severe pneumonia some alveoli are permanently replaced by scar through organisation of the exudate.
See *Pathology*, p. 69.

A62. This is vascular granulation tissue, the first stage in the organisation of an acute inflammatory exudate on the way to producing a scar, which represents complete healing. New capillaries have grown out into the area of tissue damage to form an interconnected network of new vessels; some of the macrophages and lymphocytes remaining from the later stages of inflammation lie between the capillaries.

A63. Vascular granulation tissue converts into **fibrovascular granulation tissue** by the proliferation of fibroblasts in the spaces between the capillaries. Fibrovascular granulation tissue eventually becomes **fibrous granulation tissue** by the deposition of collagen by fibroblasts; this is accompanied by progressive reduction in the number of blood vessels, until the area is largely composed of collagen, with only a few residual blood vessels remaining. This is a **fibrous scar.**
See *Pathology*, p. 70.

A64. This pattern of chronic inflammation is called **granulomatous inflammation** and has many causes worldwide.

A65. The most likely cause in this case, bearing in mind the history and the finding of multiple nodules in the lungs, together with a large cavitating abscess at the right upper lung pole, is **pulmonary tuberculosis,** due to infection by *Mycobacterium tuberculosis.*

A66. The amorphous granular pink-staining material at the centre of the lesion is called **caseous necrosis**. The arrowed giant cell is a **Langhans' giant cell**.
See *Pathology*, p. 76.

A67. A is called **the Ghon focus**.

A68. The combination of Ghon focus and tuberculous regional lymph nodes is called 'the primary complex'.

A69. The initial tuberculous lesion, the Ghon focus, and the involved lymph nodes would heal by surrounding the infected material by fibrosis, often with the deposition of calcium salts. This confines the organisms and prevents spread, and the bacteria usually die.

A70. When the child is malnourished or immunosuppressed the infection can progress, with fatal results. There is spread of organisms within the lung and other organs as a result of large caseating lymph nodes at the lung hilum eroding either bronchial wall or thin-walled blood vessels. Organisms which gain access to the bronchial tree spread down to other areas of the lung (**tuberculous bronchopneumonia**), whereas those which enter the bloodstream are widely disseminated to other organs, particularly liver, spleen and kidney, where they set up vast numbers of tiny new areas of caseating granulomatous inflammation (**miliary tuberculosis**).
See *Pathology*, p. 77.

A71. Agenesis is the name given to complete failure of organ development. **Hypoplasia** is the name given to incomplete organ development.
A72. The syndrome associated with complete renal agenesis is **Potter's syndrome**.
A73. When the fetus has Potter's syndrome, there is deficiency in amniotic fluid in which the fetus floats in the uterus. This is called **'oligohydramnios'**. A proportion of the amniotic fluid is generated by urine secreted by the fetal kidney, and this component is missing when the kidneys fail to develop.
See *Pathology*, p. 83.

A74. The name given to abnormal tissue organisation is **'dysplasia'**. Note that this word is more widely used to describe abnormal organisation and differentiation of epithelial cells on surfaces as an acquired abnormality, an important preliminary step in the development of malignant change in the epithelium (see *Pathology*, p. 44).
A75. Although the kidneys are present as structures, they are completely disorganised histologically, with no formation of cohesive functioning nephrons, so there is no renal function and hence no urine production.
A76. Because there is no urine production, there is reduction in amniotic fluid, which leads to oligohydramnios.
A77. No. Dysplasia affecting a single kidney, or a segment of an otherwise normal kidney, is much more common than total bilateral renal dysplasia. It predisposes to recurrent renal infection.
See *Pathology*, p. 83.

A78. This is a **myelomeningocele.** It is the result of failure of embryological closure of the neural tube (neural tube defect).
A79. This is frequently associated with an abnormality called the **Arnold–Chiari malformation** in which there is herniation of the cerebellum through the foramen magnum, leading to hydrocephalus (see *Pathology*, p. 420).
A80. Ultrasound scanning is a non-invasive procedure which will detect gross structural abnormalities such as that shown here. Neural crest abnormalities can also be diagnosed by the presence of large amounts of α-fetoprotein in the amniotic fluid, a sample of which is obtained by the invasive procedure of amniocentesis. This investigation is carried out after screening maternal serum for raised levels of α-fetoprotein.
See *Pathology*, p. 83.

A81. Turner's syndrome.
A82. 'Webbing'.

A83. Chromosomally, Turner's syndrome is XO (or X–). This abnormality usually arises as a result of non-disjunction during the meiotic division in gamete formation. See *Pathology*, p. 90.

A84. This is an example of cleft palate.

A85. It frequently co-exists with a structural abnormality of the upper lip called '**hare lip**' in which the upper lip is split into two portions by a vertical split.

A86. Cleft palate and hare lip are examples of failure of complete fusion of embryological primordia.

A87. Cleft palate causes great difficulty with feeding (food tending to pass into the nasal cavity) and with phonation (the palate being essential for clear precise speech). Hare lip is cosmetically unpleasing and leads to psychological disturbances. Both cleft palate and hare lip can be treated surgically, particularly if the defects are minor. See *Pathology*, p. 98.

A88. The disease shown is the tertiary stage of syphilis. Affected patients do not have all of the above manifestations; for example, patients with the cardiovascular complications rarely have a central nervous system disease, and vice versa.

A89. The causative organism is the spirochaete, *Treponema pallidum.*

A90. A gumma is a localised area of organ or tissue necrosis with a central amorphous area of necrotic tissue (resembling the caseous necrosis seen in TB), surrounded by a granulomatous reaction in which there may be giant cells of Langhans' type, lymphocytes, plasma cells and fibroblasts.

A91. The primary lesion in syphilis is the **chancre**, a firm papule which may undergo central ulceration, usually located on the genital mucosa, lips or tongue. The organism is sexually transmitted. See *Pathology*, p. 108.

A92. The dark intranuclear bodies labelled **A** are giant viral inclusion bodies within cell nuclei.

A93. The histological appearances are characteristic of CMV (cytomegalovirus) infection; the enormous size of the infected cells are the explanation for the virus being named 'cytomegalovirus'.

A94. Cytomegalovirus rarely produces significant disease unless the patient is substantially **immunosuppressed**, in this case due to immunosuppressive therapy to prevent transplant rejection. Cytomegalovirus infection is also important in AIDS. See *Pathology*, p. 110.

A95. Frostbite, producing necrosis of the toes.
A96. Localised cold injury produces vaso-constriction and thrombosis in small arteries at the periphery.
A97. Fingers, tip of the nose and the pinna may also be affected if these areas are not protected.
See *Pathology*, p. 114.

A98. The coronary artery has three small lumina instead of a single substantial lumen. This is due to **recanalisation** of old luminal thrombus.
A99. The coronary artery lumen has been occluded by a thrombus. The thrombus has undergone organisation with the development of new vessels, which have developed during the vascular granulation tissue phase and persisted. These persistent blood vessels have enlarged and established continuity through the previous blockage.
A100. At some stage before the patient died, probably many months or years before, this main coronary artery has been occluded by thrombus. Thus the patient would have evidence of a substantial old healed and fibrosed myocardial infarct, probably full thickness.
See *Pathology*, p. 125.

A101. The thromboembolus is impacted in a major pulmonary **artery**.
A102. The most common source of embolus is from the deep veins of the calf and thigh.
A103. The leg vein thrombus has become detached, passed into the iliofemoral vein, into the inferior vena cava, thence into the right atrium, right ventricle, through the pulmonary valve into the main pulmonary trunk, then into one of the major pulmonary arteries where it has become impacted because it is too big to pass any further.
A104. A thromboembolus of this size impacted in a main pulmonary vessel abruptly cuts off the blood supply to one lung, but also instantly greatly increases the peripheral resistance to the outflow of blood from the right side of the heart. This leads to **sudden death**, usually after a few minutes' acute breathlessness, cyanosis and collapse, due to acute right heart failure.
See *Pathology*, p. 126.

A105. The lesion labelled **A** is an established **renal infarct**, probably 5–10 days'old, resulting from abrupt occlusion of a branch renal artery to the upper pole.
A106. This is most likely due to a thromboembolus arising from the left side of the heart. In view of the history of angina and recent myocardial infarction, the probable cause is a **mural throm-**

bus formed on the wall of the left ventricle damaged by recent myocardial infarction. Other possible causes are thrombotic vegetations on the heart valves, or a thrombus in the auricular appendage of the left atrium.

A107. The pale area will show necrotic kidney, although the ghost of glomerular and tubular structures will still be visible. This is an example of **coagulative necrosis**.

A108. The hemiplegia is almost certainly due to a thromboembolus from the left ventricle. The thromboembolus has passed into the relevant cerebral artery to produce cerebral infarction. Other sites particularly prone to infarction following embolism from mural thrombus include the spleen and small intestine.
See *Pathology*, p. 128.

A109. This is a **purpuric** skin rash.

A110. The confluent small red blotches are produced because of leakage of red cells from damaged blood vessels (mainly venules) in the dermis. This is usually due to destructive inflammation of the vessel walls (**vasculitis**).

A111. Vasculitic purpuric skin rashes can have many causes: drugs are an important one and, in this case, the most likely cause as the patient is receiving drug therapy for rheumatoid disease. However, vasculitic skin rashes can also occur as a component of autoimmune connective tissue diseases, including rheumatoid disease and systemic vasculitis.
See *Pathology*, p. 139.

A112. The lesion is a full-thickness regional infarction of the lateral wall of the left ventricle.

A113. It is composed of pale necrotic tissue with a surrounding rim of hyperaemia, and is probably 7–10 days' old.

A114. The lesion is full-thickness (i.e. involving pericardium, myocardium and endocardium) and is located in the lateral wall of the left ventricle. The abnormality also present would be an occlusion of the circumflex branch of the left coronary artery; the occlusion would most likely be a thrombus obliterating a lumen already reduced by atheroma. A bleed into an atheromatous plaque is another possibility.
See *Pathology*, p. 145.

A115. Haemopericardium.

A116. Distension of the pericardial cavity with blood leads to **cardiac tamponade**, acute cardiac failure due to inability of the atria to fill, resulting from the high external pressure in the pericardial cavity.

A117. The most likely cause is **rupture** of a full-thickness myocardial infarct, shown in the partly blood-filled track to the left of the label (**A**). This complication of myocardial infarct is most likely to occur between 4 and 10 days after infarction, at which time the damaged wall is at its weakest because of advanced macrophage removal of necrotic tissue.

A118. Although haemopericardium can be traumatic (e.g. following chest injuries in a vehicular accident) the other common spontaneous cause is **dissecting aneurysm** of the ascending aorta with retrograde spread of blood into pericardial cavity.
See *Pathology*, p. 148.

A119. The lesion labelled (**A**) is a **mural thrombus**, formed over the area of endocardium damaged by myocardial infarction.
A120. **Cardiac dysrhythmia; acute left ventricular failure; rupture of ventricular wall through infarcted area (see Q115–118); papillary muscle dysfunction or infarction; acute pericarditis.**
A121. The dense hemiplegia is due to embolisation of thrombotic material from the mural thrombus into a major cerebral artery.
See *Pathology*, p. 148.

A122. The abnormality is a **ventricular aneurysm**, aneurysmal bulging of the left ventricular wall made thin and non-contractile by the replacement of necrotic muscle by rigid but inelastic fibrous scar.
A123. The long-term complications of myocardial infarct are: **further episodes of myocardial infarction (because of the severity of the underlying coronary artery insufficiency); chronic intractable heart failure (due to inadequate left ventricular pumping action).** Dressler's syndrome is a form of immune mediated pericarditis associated with a high ESR, occurring 2–10 months after an acute myocardial infarct. It is rare.
See *Pathology*, p. 149.

A124. The structure labelled (**A**) is called 'a vegetation'—a mass of thrombotic material deposited on a heart valve, usually a mitral or aortic valve.
A125. As a thrombus, it is composed of aggregated masses of platelets and fibrin, with entrapped red and white cells. If it is an infected thrombus (by bacteria or fungi), organisms and large numbers of neutrophil polymorphs will also be present.
A126. The commonest type of valve vegetation is the '**marantic**' vegetation, composed entirely of thrombus, with no associated infection; this is usually a terminal event in patients with widespread cancer. Infected vegetations (infective endocarditis) are of three types: **subacute bacterial endocarditis,** in which the infected thrombotic vegetation occurs on valves previously damaged by some other disease, usually rheumatic endocarditis; **acute bacterial endocarditis**, which occurs as a complication of bacteraemia due to virulent organisms and can occur on previously normal valves; and

fungal endocarditis, usually due to *Candida,* which also occurs on previously normal heart valves.

A127. Acute bacterial endocarditis destroys the valve, leading to acute cardiac failure from valve incompetence. Subacute bacterial endocarditis does not destroy the valve, but causes illness and death from multiple embolic episodes, with fragments of the vegetation breaking off and entering the systemic circulation. Marantic vegetations behave in a similar manner.
See *Pathology,* p. 152.

A128. The disease is **mitral stenosis,** resulting from chronic rheumatic endocarditis. Mitral stenosis leads to chronic thickening and fusion of the normally thin mobile mitral valve leaflets associated with thickening and fusion of the chordae tendinae, which tether the leaflets to the ventricular wall.

A129. The patient has had **rheumatic fever** as a child, with a pancarditis (pericarditis, myocarditis and endocarditis). Fibrous healing of the inflamed mitral valve has led to progressive thickening, distortion and fusion over a period of many years.

A130. The mitral valve is unable to open during diastole (leading to functional stenosis), and will also be unable to close fully during systole (leading to mitral incompetence). Both of these will lead to increased pressure in the left atrium, which will become greatly distended, and the rise in pressure in the left atrium will be reflected back along the pulmonary veins and into the pulmonary capillary bed, leading to a tendency to **pulmonary capillary congestion** and **pulmonary oedema.** At the same time, the output of the left ventricle may be reduced. This leads to left ventricular failure and, eventually, secondary right heart failure (**congestive cardiac failure**).

A131. The other commonly involved valve in chronic rheumatic endocarditis is the aortic valve, which may become similarly thickened, fused and stenotic or incompetent.
See *Pathology,* p. 152.

A132. This is **mitral valve prolapse** or **floppy valve syndrome.** It is particularly common in young adults, mainly women.

A133. The valve leaflet becomes degenerate, with the rigid central zona fibrosa undergoing myxoid degeneration, leading to softening of the valves, which then bulge upwards during diastole, particularly the posterior mitral valve leaflet.

A134. The increased mobility of the valve leaflets frequently leads to a mild degree of mitral valve incompetence during systole. A severe complication is the sudden onset of acute cardiac failure due to rupture of one of the chordae tendinae tethering the hypermobile leaflet, the increased mobility leading to a tendency for one of the chordae to snap.
See *Pathology,* p. 153.

A135. The aortic valve leaflets (of which there appear to be only two instead of the more normal three) are greatly thickened and fused and contain large irregular nodules of calcium.

A136. This is **calcific aortic stenosis** in a **congenitally bicuspid aortic valve.**

A137. Similar fibrous thickening, calcification and fusion can occur in **chronic rheumatic endocarditis** affecting the aortic valve, although the valve is usually identifiably normally three-cusped.

A138. The aortic valve is **stenotic**, reducing the blood flow through the valve into the aorta and systemic circulation during systole. As a result there is a low pulse pressure (difference between systolic and diastolic pressures), and hypoperfusion of organs may occur; for example, the patient may suffer 'black-outs' due to hypoperfusion of the brain, and there may be ischaemia of the myocardium because of poor coronary artery flow. Because the left ventricle has to strain to force blood out through the blocked valve, there is marked **left ventricular hypertrophy.**
See *Pathology*, p. 153.

A139. The four features are:
A **ventricular septal defect (VSD).**
An **overriding aorta** (sits astride the VSD so that it receives blood from both right and left ventricles).
Pulmonary outflow tract stenosis, either valvar or sub-valvar.
Right ventricular hypertrophy.

A140. The ventricular septal defect, combined with the high pressure in the hypertrophied right ventricle, leads to some shunting of deoxygenated blood from the right side of the heart to the left **(right-to-left shunt).** The mixed oxygenated and deoxygenated blood from the left and right ventricles passes into the systemic circulation through the overriding aorta, so that there is **cyanosis.** Much of the right ventricular output of blood enters the systemic circulation in this way, and very little passes through the stenotic pulmonary outflow, so the lungs are very poorly perfused with deoxygenated blood, and oxygenation is further impaired.

A141. Surgical correction is aimed at:
Relieving pulmonary outflow stenosis, to allow adequate lung perfusion.
Closing the ventricular septal defect, to prevent right-to-left shunt.
Rechannelling the flow, so that the aorta receives blood only from the left ventricle.
See *Pathology*, p. 156.

A142. A = alveoli of lung. **B** = bronchiole.

A143. The purplish-staining material filling the alveoli and bronchiole is **pus**, an acute inflammatory exudate rich in neutrophils.

A144. The disease is **bronchopneumonia,** a bacterial infection of the lung in which the bacteria gain access to the lung by spreading down the tracheobronchial tree from an infection in the upper respiratory tract.
A145. His **age,** his **immobility** and his **unconscious state.** This pattern of disease, which is most common in infancy and old age, is predisposed by the presence of debility and immobility. Patients who are immobile develop retention of secretions; these gravitate to the dependent parts of the lungs and become infected—hence, bronchopneumonia most commonly involves the lower lobes.
See *Pathology,* p. 163.

A146. His chest pain is due to **acute pleurisy**, characteristically a sharp jabbing pain occurring in time with breathing and coughing.
A147. His underlying lung disease is **lobar pneumonia,** extensive consolidation of (in this case) the right upper and lower lobes by pneumonic consolidation.
A148. The material labelled **A** on the surface of the upper and lower lobes is an acute inflammatory exudate rich in fibrin.
A149. The main physical sign on auscultation of the lung will be a harsh scratching noise synchronous with breathing and coughing. This is called a **pleural friction rub**, and is due to the noise made by the fibrinous exudate over the lung rubbing against the parietal pleura. Consolidation of the lung due to pneumonia may also manifest as bronchial breathing and poor air entry.
See *Pathology,* p. 164.

A150. A are abnormally dilated and thick-walled bronchial air passages extending out to the lung periphery.
A151. The disease is **chronic bronchiectasis**.
A152. The two main factors in the pathogenesis of bronchiectasis are:
> **Interference with drainage of bronchial secretions.**
> **Persistent infection weakening the bronchial walls.**

A153. Complications include: chronic suppuration, lung abscess, blood-borne spread of infection (often leading to brain abscess), and development of generalised amyloidosis after a long history.
See *Pathology,* p. 167.

A154. A is thick mucus, often containing eosinophil leucocytes and their products, obliterating the bronchial lumen.
A155. B labels the hypertrophied smooth muscle in the bronchial wall, an important factor in narrowing the bronchus by bronchospasm.
A156. Type I hypersensitivity reaction.
A157. Chronic obstructive airways disease (COAD).
See *Pathology,* p. 169.

A158. The other common pattern of generalised emphysema is **panacinar emphysema**.

A159. In centriacinar emphysema, the dilated air spaces are the respiratory bronchioles.

A160. In panacinar emphysema there is dilatation of terminal alveoli, alveolar ducts and respiratory bronchioles. See *Pathology*, p. 171.

A161. This appearance is called 'honeycomb lung'.

A162. Histologically, there is coalescence of air spaces, both alveoli, alveolar ducts and bronchioles, to form large cystic spaces lined with cuboidal and sometimes respiratory or squamous epithelium, surrounded by fibrosis and proliferated smooth muscle. See *Pathology*, p. 176.

A163. The areas labelled **A** are composed of dense hyaline collagenous tissue and macrophages, containing large numbers of small silicon particles.

A164. The areas are black because they contain large quantities of carbon inhaled with the silica.

A165. The patient was a coal miner working in a coal seam where the coal has a high silica content. See *Pathology*, p. 178.

A166. The brown material is a collection of **asbestos bodies**, formed by the deposition of haemosiderin-containing protein around long asbestos fibres. The asbestos gains access to the lung air spaces by inhalation in an atmosphere in which asbestos fibres are circulating. In this case, the presence of asbestos has stimulated pulmonary fibrosis.

A167. Other disorders associated with inhalation of asbestos are the malignant tumour of the pleura, **malignant mesothelioma**, and thick collagenous fibrous pleural plaques, often producing recurrent pleural effusions. Asbestos exposure also predisposes to carcinoma of the lung. The progressive pulmonary fibrosis due to asbestos inhalation is called **asbestosis.**

A168. Yes. The occupation of a lagger in a shipyard involved packing asbestos insulation around pipes. See *Pathology*, p. 179.

A169. The photograph shows a carcinoma arising in a lower lobe bronchus, with spread to peribronchial lymph nodes.

A170. The most likely histological pattern is squamous cell carcinoma (50%), although the tumour may also be an anaplastic carcinoma of small or large cell type (30%). Adenocarcinoma rarely arises near the hilum in a major bronchus.

A171. Haemoptysis is due to ulceration by tumour of the bronchial mucosa.

A172. The recurrent infections are almost certainly due to inability to clear bronchial secretions through the greatly narrowed tumorous lower lobe bronchus.
See *Pathology*, p. 181.

A173. This is most likely a **peripheral carcinoma of the lung**.
A174. Most peripheral lung cancers are **adenocarcinomas**.
A175. This tumour has arisen in a small area of previous lung scarring ('scar cancer'). Smoking is not such an important aetiological factor in adenocarcinoma as it is in the other forms of bronchial and lung cancer.
A176. Peripheral adenocarcinomas, particularly scar cancers, can metastasise widely, as in this case, and the primary tumour often remains small.
See *Pathology*, p. 181.

A177. The lesion is an ulcerating **squamous cell carcinoma** of the lower lip.
A178. The tumour spreads by local invasion and via lymphatics to regional lymph nodes in the neck.
A179. The lower lip is the commonest site for squamous cell carcinoma in the mouth: the tongue (the lateral border of the anterior two-thirds) is the second most common site. The floor of the mouth and the cheek are less common sites in the UK and USA but are more common in the Indian subcontinent.
See *Pathology*, p. 197.

A180. The lesion is in the **parotid salivary gland**.
A181. The most likely diagnosis is **pleomorphic salivary adenoma**, a slow-growing benign tumour.
A182. Surgical excision is hampered by the fact that the facial nerve runs through the parotid gland, and may be damaged in attempts at complete removal of the tumour. Although the tumour is benign, incomplete removal may be followed by regrowth of the tumour.
A183. Other possibilities are Warthin's tumour (which is benign), adenoid cystic carcinoma, and muco-epidermoid carcinoma (both of which are malignant tumours).
See *Pathology*, p. 198.

A184. This is a **basal cell carcinoma**, arising on the skin of the nose. The head and neck are the most important sites for this tumour.
A185. Yes. Most basal cell carcinomas arise as small nodules that undergo central ulceration and have raised pearly/white edges.

A186. The tumours are malignant in that they are invasive and, if neglected, can lead to extensive local tissue destruction ('rodent ulcer'). They do not metastasise to distant sites.
A187. The most important aetiological factor is prolonged unprotected exposure to sunlight.
See *Pathology*, p. 204.

A188. The red arrow points to enlarged lymph nodes in the neck, the enlargement being due to metastatic carcinoma of the nasopharynx. This is an important and common presenting feature of this tumour.
A189. Obstruction to the Eustachian tube by the tumour prevents drainage of fluid from the middle ear, and leads to **secretory otitis media**; this may result in hearing loss and tinnitus.
See *Pathology*, p. 207.

A190. The irregular white mass is a **cholesteatoma**.
A191. Histologically, it resembles an epidermoid cyst, being lined by flattened keratinising squamous epithelium and filled with masses of keratin, the white material which can be seen in the picture.
A192. The main complications are continuing infection of the middle ear, with the risk of brain abscess; mastoiditis and meningitis; and progressive expansion of the cholesteatoma, eroding the bone of the skull. This erosion may destroy the labyrinth, the facial nerve and the mastoid air cells, and may occasionally erode through the skull into the middle cranial fossa of the brain.
See *Pathology*, p. 210.

A193. The structure labelled **A** is an **invasive squamous cell carcinoma of the larynx**.
A194. The most likely presenting symptom is **loss of voice**, but in an advanced neglected lesion like this, the lumen of the larynx may be greatly reduced, leading to **stridor**.
A195. Carcinomas of the larynx can be classified by location:
   • Supraglottic carcinoma (in the aryepiglottic folds, false cords and ventricles).
   • Glottic carcinoma (in the true vocal cords and anterior and posterior commissures).
   • Subglottic carcinoma (below the true vocal cords and above the first tracheal ring).
Glottic carcinomas have the best prognosis because they present earliest, have a poor lymphatic drainage, and may present and be resected before spread has occurred. The other two types have a worse prognosis because of later presentation and a more abundant lymphatic drainage.

A196. Spread is by local invasion and lymphatic spread to lymph nodes in the neck.
See *Pathology,* p. 215.

A197. C indicates the oesophago–gastric junction, where under normal circumstances the squamous mucosa of the oesophagus would change to the columnar epithelium of the stomach. **A** indicates the lower oesophageal mucosa which, in Barrett's oesophagus, is of columnar cells resembling gastric mucosa. **B** indicates multiple ulcers in the abnormal mucosa.
A198. Persistent oesophageal reflux causes metaplasia of the lower oesophageal mucosa, the normal oesophageal squamous epithelium being replaced by glandular epithelium.
A199. Complications of Barrett's oesophagus are:
• Predisposition to recurrent peptic ulceration, often leading to eventual fibrous stricture.
• Predisposition to the development of adenocarcinoma in the lower oesophagus arising from the metaplastic glandular epithelium. This usually follows a period of severe dysplasia in the abnormal glandular epithelium.
See *Pathology,* p. 218.

A200. The stomach mucosa shows **acute erosive gastritis,** with multiple superficial haemorrhagic areas of mucosal loss ('erosions') and a small superficial ulcer.
A201. This may be produced by acute shock; stress associated with raised intracranial pressure or severe burns; certain drugs, particularly aspirin and non-steroidal anti-inflammatory agents; and heavy acute alcohol ingestion.
A202. In this man's case there are two possible causes—acute alcohol ingestion and drugs. He was probably receiving non-steroidal anti-inflammatory drugs for his ankylosing spondylitis.
See *Pathology,* p. 221.

A203. The lesion is a large benign chronic peptic ulcer.
A204. Peptic ulceration arises because of breakdown of the normal mechanisms which protect the mucosa against acid attack. In the stomach the most important factors are:
• Surface epithelial damage caused by *Helicobacter pylori* infection.
• Toxic damage to surface epithelium by non-steroidal anti-inflammatory drugs.
• Bile regurgitation due to incompetence of the pylorus.
Chronic gastritis and smoking are also believed to play a role.
A205. The important complications are:
• Haemorrhage from an eroded vessel in the floor of the ulcer, leading to haematemesis.
• Perforation, leading to peritonitis.

• Penetration, in which the ulcer penetrates the full-thickness of the stomach wall and adheres to adjacent organs, such as the liver or pancreas, which are then damaged by continuing penetration.

• Pyloric stenosis, due to fibrous stricture from the fibrous healing attempts.

See *Pathology*, p. 222.

A206. (a) is from the normal child; (b) is from the child who is failing to thrive.

A207. The abnormal jejunal mucosa is perfectly flat and shows none of the raised villous pattern of the mucosa seen in the normal child. This flattening, which is due to **total villous atrophy**, leads to a great reduction in the absorptive surface area.

A208. The most likely diagnosis in a child is **coeliac disease**.

A209. Coeliac disease (gluten enteropathy) is due to abnormal immune sensitivity to the protein gliadin, a component of the wheat flour protein, gluten. Immune damage to the mucosa leads to villous atrophy, which is potentially recoverable if gluten is removed from the diet.

See *Pathology*, p. 227.

A210. The area labelled **A** shows marked thickening of the bowel wall, mainly due to submucosal thickening, associated with inflammation throughout all layers of the wall, and fissured ulceration of the mucosa.

A211. The most likely diagnosis is Crohn's disease.

A212. Crohn's disease may involve anywhere in the alimentary tract, from the mouth, where it presents with a swollen and oedematous mucosa with fissured ulcers, to the anus, where it often manifests with fistulae.

A213. The main direct complications of Crohn's disease are:

• Stricture formation and fibrous adhesions.

• Perforation of the bowel.

• Perianal fistulae, fissures and abscesses.

See *Pathology*, p. 228.

A214. Ulcerative colitis (active).

A215. In ulcerative colitis, ulceration is superficial but usually very extensive, leading to massive loss of absorptive mucosa. In Crohn's disease, the ulcers are deep and fissured.

A216. Ulcerative colitis is a chronic remitting disease with active acute, chronic quiescent and fulminant active patterns. Approximately 80% of patients have chronic quiescent disease, with infrequent episodes of relapse; 10% have persistent active disease, despite treatment; and 10% have severe disease, requiring early surgery.

A217. The most important indications are to **patient request**, because of inability to cope with active severe symptomatic disease not responding to medical therapy; **fulminant active disease**, leading to the life-threatening condition of acute toxic megacolon; and **long-standing chronic active disease** (over 10 years' duration), because of the risks of malignancy in this group. The development of invasive adenocarcinoma is usually preceded by development of dysplastic changes in the colonic epithelium.
See *Pathology*, p. 229.

A218. Both are patterns of colonic adenoma: (a) is a typical tubular adenoma; (b) is a typical villous adenoma.
A219. Tubular adenomas are characteristically pedunculated, with the tumour **A** in (a) being located on a stalk (**B**) composed of normal colonic mucosa. Villous adenomas are sessile, arising from a broad base.
A220. Both types may cause bleeding per rectum and the most important complication in both patterns is malignant change to form adenocarcinomas.
See *Pathology*, p. 231.

A221. The lesion labelled is an adenocarcinoma of the colon—here, the sigmoid colon.
A222. In the sigmoid colon, the most common presenting symptom is alteration of bowel habit and passing blood per rectum. In the caecum and right colon, tumours reach a larger size before presenting and may present with anaemia due to chronic blood loss or obstruction.
A223. The main spread is by local invasion through the bowel wall to involve the adjacent structures, lymphatic spread to regional lymph nodes, and bloodstream spread via the portal vein to the liver.
A224. The main prognostic features are depth of invasion through the colon wall and presence of lymph node metastases (Dukes staging—see *Pathology*, p. 234) and the presence of tumour in blood vessels.
See *Pathology*, p. 233.

A225. The discoloured area is the result of **small bowel infarction**.
A226. The three main causes are:
• Arterial infarction due to **emboli from intracardiac thrombosis**—for example, mural thrombus on a myocardial infarct.
• Arterial infarction due to **thrombosis in the mesenteric artery**, which is partly occluded by atherosclerosis. This is an important cause in patients with generalised atherosclerosis.
• Venous infarction due to strangulation—e.g. entrapment of a loop of bowel in a tight hernial sac or volvulus.

A227. In this man with severe heart disease the most likely cause is embolus from intracardiac thrombosis, but he will probably have severe atherosclerosis in vessels other than coronary arteries so there may be thrombosis of the mesenteric artery.
See *Pathology*, p. 235.

A228. Meconium ileus is an important manifestation and presentation of the autosomal recessive disorder, **cystic fibrosis.**
A229. The pancreatic feature of cystic fibrosis is **malabsorption,** due to failure of the exocrine pancreas to produce digestive enzymes, the result of long-term obliteration of pancreatic ducts by thick mucus.
The pulmonary features of cystic fibrosis are **bronchiectasis** and recurrent **chest infection** due to thick mucus in the bronchial tree.
See *Pathology*, p. 240.

A230. The yellow colour is due to excessive fat deposition in the liver cells.
A231. Histologically, the liver will show extensive fatty change, with large numbers of lipid droplets within hepatocytes. In addition, there may be extensive liver cell necrosis, depending on the cause of the fatty change.
A232. Fatty change can be due to:
   • Metabolic stress, including diabetes mellitus or severe malnutrition.
   • Toxins, particularly alcohol.
It may also occur in pregnancy and in infants (Reye's syndrome).
In this case, acute alcoholic hepatitis is the most likely cause.
A233. In addition to metabolic fatty change, a yellow liver may be due to extensive acute liver cell necrosis due to viral infection ('acute yellow atrophy') and extensive liver cell necrosis due to drugs—for example, paracetamol.
See *Pathology*, p. 246.

A234. The lesions labelled **A** are multiple **liver abscesses**.
A235. The three main routes by which bacteria enter the liver are:
   • Ascending spread from the duodenum via the biliary tree **(ascending cholangitis).**
   • Spread from the alimentary tract through the hepatic portal venous system **(portal pyaemia).**
   • Bloodstream spread by the hepatic artery as part of a systemic septicaemia.
A236. The non-invasive methods of imaging these lesions are ultrasound and CT scan. The lesions can be sampled by needle biopsy, with material being sent for microbiological culture.
See *Pathology*, p. 253.

A237. This irregular nodularity of the liver is due to **cirrhosis**.
A238. The three key histological features are:
• Long-standing widespread destruction of liver cells.
• Fibrosis leading to interlinked bands throughout the liver.
• Regenerative nodules of new liver cells which are, however, not linked in the normal way to the vascular system and bile ducts.
A239. The most likely cause of her massive haematemesis is bleeding from **oesophageal varices**. Destruction of the liver architecture leads to blockage of the intrahepatic branches of the portal venous system, leading to raised portal venous pressure (**portal hypertension**). This high pressure leads to opening up of anastomoses between the portal and systemic venous system, the most important site being beneath the mucosa in the lower oesophagus. These distended anastomoses protrude into the oesophageal lumen, protected only by mucosa, and are easily eroded to produce torrential haemorrhage.
See *Pathology*, p. 259.

A240. The scattered white, partly necrotic, areas labelled **A** in the cirrhotic liver are malignant tumours, **primary hepatocellular carcinoma**.
A241. The predisposing factors are:
• Hepatic cirrhosis of whatever cause.
• Hepatitis B infection with chronic carrier status.
• Toxins in food—for example the mycotoxin from the fungus *Aspergillus flavus,* a frequent contaminant of stored nuts and grains in tropical countries.
A242. The serum α-fetoprotein level, which is raised in cases of primary hepatocellular carcinoma, may be used as a tumour marker.
See *Pathology*, p. 263.

A243. Photograph (a) shows **cholesterol stones**, in which the major component is cholesterol (mixed with calcium salts and small amounts of bilirubin). They form when bile becomes supersaturated with cholesterol because there are insufficient bile salts to keep the cholesterol in solution.
A244. The gallstones in (b) are typical **pigment stones**, with a high proportion of bilirubin and calcium salts but very little cholesterol. The most important predisposing factor to pigment stone formation is abnormally high red cell breakdown in the spleen such as may occur in chronic haemolytic anaemias, resulting in greatly increased bilirubin production.
A245. The presence of gallstones may lead to mucosal ulceration by friction in the gallbladder. If stones become impacted in the neck of the gallbladder or cystic duct, flow of bile out of the gallbladder is obstructed; attempts to force bile out lead to marked hypertrophy of the gallbladder muscle wall with diverticulum for-

mation, mucosa being forced in pouches into the gallbladder wall
(Aschoff–Rokitansky sinuses). These changes are commonly called
'chronic cholecystitis'.
A246. Yes. Carcinoma of the gallbladder is usually associated with
gallstones and 'chronic cholecystitis'.
See *Pathology*, p. 265 and 266.

A247. Acute necrotising pancreatitis.
A248. The areas labelled **B** are foci of **fat necrosis** caused by leakage of lipase enzymes from the dying exocrine pancreas cells, producing local destruction of triglycerides in local adipose tissue.
A249. The **serum amylase** would have been greatly raised, having
leaked from the dying pancreatic exocrine cells into the blood circulation.
A250. The most likely predisposing factor in a patient of this age
and with his social history is **alcohol consumption**.
See *Pathology*, p. 268.

A251. The lesion marked **A** in the head of the pancreas is a homogeneous mass replacing the normal lobular pattern of the pancreas, and is an **adenocarcinoma**.
A252. Carcinomas in the head of the pancreas tend to present
with **obstructive jaundice**, due to obstruction of the distal bile duct
as it passes through the head of the pancreas. There may also be
chronic back pain associated with weight loss and anorexia. Rarely,
the patient may develop multiple venous thromboses in leg veins.
A253. The prognosis for carcinoma of the pancreas is extremely
poor: 90% of patients die within 6 months of diagnosis.
See *Pathology*, p. 268.

A254. The well-circumscribed creamy white masses are homoge-
neously enlarged cervical lymph nodes.
A255. The possibilities are reactive lymph node hyperplasia,
metastatic tumour in lymph nodes, primary malignant lymphoma
and leukaemic infiltration of lymph nodes.
A256. Because there are probably similar masses in the axillae and
inguinal lymph node regions, the most likely diagnosis is **primary
malignant lymphoma**, either Hodgkin's disease or non-Hodgkin's
lymphoma.
A257. The only way to establish an accurate diagnosis is **histological examination** of an abnormal lymph node.
See *Pathology*, p. 274.

A258. The cell is a classical binucleate Reed–Sternberg cell.
A259. Reed–Sternberg cells are characteristic of **Hodgkin's
disease**.
A260. Hodgkin's disease can be classified into four main types,

according to histological appearances (Rye classification):
- Lymphocyte-predominant Hodgkin's disease (10%).
- Mixed cellularity Hodgkin's disease (20%).
- Nodular sclerosis Types I and II Hodgkin's disease (60–70%).
- Lymphocyte-depleted Hodgkin's disease (less than 5%).

Lymphocyte-predominant Hodgkin's disease has the best prognosis and lymphocyte-depleted Hodgkin's disease the poorest prognosis. See *Pathology*, p. 276.

A261. The most likely diagnosis is non-Hodgkin's lymphoma. The actual type is small-cell lymphocytic B-cell lymphoma. Learning the various classifications of non-Hodgkin's lymphomas is something not to be undertaken lightly and you will need to be very strong!

A262. The most likely cause of his anaemia is bone marrow replacement by the same type of malignant lymphocytes, leading to impaired production of red blood cells.

A263. Elderly patients with this type of lymphoma frequently have some degree of immune deficiency associated with hypogamma-globinaemia, and are prone to recurrent severe infections.

A264. Despite the haematological and infective complications, the prognosis of this type is good, with a 5-year survival rate greater than 60%.
See *Pathology*, p. 280.

A265. The bone marrow is abnormal because the normal fatty and haemopoietic marrow has been completely destroyed and replaced by masses of abnormal white cell precursors, uniformly filling the marrow spaces.

A266. The most likely diagnosis is some form of **leukaemia**—a malignant proliferation of white cell precursors in the bone mar-row—destroying normal erythropoietic cells (hence the anaemia), megakaryocytes (hence the thrombocytopenia) and normal mature functioning white cells, particularly neutrophil polymorphs (neutropenia).

A267. High-magnification light microscopy of the white cells circulat-ing in the peripheral blood, white cells obtained from the bone mar-row by aspiration, and the leukaemic cells obtained, as in this photomicrograph by trephine biopsy. These studies will indicate whether the leukaemia is acute or chronic, and whether the leukae-mic cells belong to the lymphocyte line or the myeloid/monocytic line.
See *Pathology*, p. 292.

A268. The cells replacing normal haemopoietic marrow are **abnor-mal plasma cells**.

A269. The diagnosis is the plasma cell neoplasm called **multiple myeloma**.

A270. Leukoerythroblastic anaemia is caused whenever some abnormal infiltration of the bone marrow destroys normal red cell, neutrophil and platelet formation; in this case it is the malignant plasma cells which are destroying normal haemopoiesis.

A271. The proteinuria may be due to two effects:

• Patients with myeloma have a high incidence of **renal amyloid**, leading to excessive protein loss from amyloid-affected glomeruli.

• Plasma cells in myeloma secrete large amounts of monoclonal immunoglobulin, and there is often an excess of free light chains; these comparatively small molecules may be removed from the blood by the glomerulus, to pass out in the urine (Bence-Jones protein). See *Pathology*, p. 296.

A272. The lesion marked **A** is a large pituitary adenoma.

A273. His visual defect is due to compression of the optic chiasm by the enlarging tumour extending out of the pituitary fossa. In the CT scan, the stretched optic chiasm is indicated by a black arrow.

A274. This pituitary tumour was not producing any hormone secretion ('non-functioning adenoma'), but a proportion of tumours secrete anterior pituitary hormones, particularly growth hormone, ACTH and prolactin (functioning adenoma).

A275. Goliath, who was killed by David, was probably an acromegalic giant due to a growth hormone secreting pituitary adenoma. It has been speculated that his tumour was so large that it compressed the optic chiasm and produced bitemporal hemianopia; this would have restricted his field of vision greatly, enabling David to get in a sneak shot with a sling, and kill him (*The Holy Bible*, I Samuel, **17**: 1–46). See *Pathology*, p. 299.

A276. The thyroid shows enlargement due to **multinodular goitre**.

A277. Although some of the brown material is due to haemorrhage, in most cases it is translucent and gelatinous, and is **thyroid colloid**, which is stored in excess. This material is brown because of the iodine content of the thyroid colloid.

A278. Occasionally, one of the nodules in multinodular goitre is functionally as well as structurally hyperplastic, producing excess amounts of thyroid hormone, which leads to the symptoms of thyrotoxicosis; this can be an indication for surgical resection. Some multinodular goitres have a particularly large extension (often from the isthmus in the midline), which passes behind the manubrium and continues to expand in the upper anterior mediastinum. This may lead to **tracheal compression**, necessitating surgical removal. Such a goitre is called a **retrosternal goitre**. See *Pathology*, p. 301.

A279. This patient has Graves' disease, a form of autoimmune thyroiditis.

A280. There is diffuse thyroid acinar hyperplasia with increased production of thyroid hormone, leading to clinical thyrotoxicosis (hyperthyroidism).

A281. Graves' disease is an organ-specific autoimmune disease that results from the presence of an IgG antibody called the long-acting thyroid stimulator (LATS). This antibody acts directly on thyroid cells, producing hyperplasia and continuous thyroid hormone secretion, out of the feedback control of TSH from the pituitary gland.

A282. Exophthalmos—protruberant, staring eyes due to expansion of retro-orbital soft tissue, mainly expansion of orbital adipose tissue.

See *Pathology*, p. 303.

A283. The fleshy lobulated white cut surface appearance is characteristic of **Hashimoto's thyroiditis**, an organ-specific autoimmune disease.

A284. The normal thyroid acinar structure, which appears brown because of the iodine content of stored colloid, is destroyed by the autoimmune process; the white colour is largely due to heavy lymphocytic infiltrate.

A285. Apart from tests to measure thyroid function, Hashimoto's disease is characterised by the presence of an anti-microsomal antibody and an antibody against thyroglobulin.

A286. Initially, the patient may have hyperthyroidism but, in the long term, thyroid function fails as the acini are destroyed by the autoimmune process, and patients become progressively hypothyroid.

See *Pathology*, p. 304.

A287. Stridor was the result of compression of the trachea by the rapidly enlarging mass in the neck.

A288. The lump in the neck is most likely to be due to **anaplastic carcinoma of the thyroid**.

A289. Anaplastic carcinoma characteristically occurs in the elderly, and behaves in a highly malignant fashion, growing rapidly and compressing and infiltrating adjacent structures such as the trachea and jugular vein. The other main forms of thyroid carcinoma (papillary carcinoma and follicular carcinoma) are much less aggressive locally.

See *Pathology*, p. 306.

A290. The adrenals show extensive acute haemorrhagic necrosis.

A291. This syndrome is known as the 'Waterhouse–Friderichsen syndrome'—there is hypovolaemic and hypotensive shock associated with massive adrenal necrosis, the necrosis being due to vessel occlusion because of disseminated intravascular coagulation.

A292. The most likely cause is **meningococcal septicaemia**.

A293. The most important skin manifestation of meningococcal septicaemia is a widespread petechial and ecchymotic vasculitic skin rash of sudden onset (spotted fever).
See *Pathology*, p. 311.

A294. The tumour is a **neuroblastoma** derived from primitive neuroblasts in the adrenal medulla.

A295. These tumours characteristically metastasise via the bloodstream to bone and bone marrow (in particular, the bones of the face and skull are frequently involved), but also frequently spread to the lungs and liver.

A296. In addition to using imaging methods to visualise the tumour and metastases, the most important investigation is the measurement of the tumour markers—vanilylmandelic acid (VMA) and homovanillic acid (HVA)—for neuroblastoma. These are breakdown products of catecholamines that are invariably secreted by neuroblastoma. Certain diagnosis must be based on histological examination of a primary or metastatic tumour.
See *Pathology*, p. 316.

A297. A is the abdominal aorta. Its surface is roughened and irregular because of severe **atherosclerosis**.

A298. The kidney labelled **B** is smaller than normal because it has undergone chronic atrophy due to ischaemia, probably the result of stenosis of the renal artery on that side by severe atherosclerosis affecting its ostium where it originates from the aorta. The kidney on the other side is larger than normal because it is showing **compensatory hypertrophy**.

A299. The ischaemic kidney can precipitate **systemic hypertension** because of over-secretion of renin. This is one of the surgically-treatable causes of systemic hypertension. Cerebral haemorrhage in the basal ganglia region is a common and important complication of systemic hypertension.
See *Pathology*, p. 321.

A300. The disease involves only one segment of the glomerulus, and this pattern of glomerular abnormality is called **segmental** (cf global—see below).

A301. Global means the disease affects the whole of the glomerulus uniformly (cf segmental—see above).

Diffuse means affecting all glomeruli in both kidneys (cf focal).

Focal means affecting only a proportion of glomeruli, with the others completely unaffected.

Generally, primary glomerular diseases are either global and diffuse, or focal and segmental.
See *Pathology*, p. 324.

A302. The child has the **acute nephritic syndrome.**
A303. The capillary lumina are occluded by proliferating endothelial cells and some neutrophil polymorphs.
A304. This glomerular lesion is known as **acute diffuse proliferative glomerulonephritis**, and affects all parts of all glomeruli (i.e. it is global and diffuse). The proliferation occurs in association with deposition of immune complexes at the glomerular basement membrane. The immune complexes develop as a response to infection of the throat by certain strains of streptococci.
A305. In the great majority of cases in childhood acute proliferative glomerulonephritis resolves completely, leaving no permanent renal impairment.
See *Pathology*, p. 326.

A306. This patient has the **nephrotic syndrome.**
A307. The nephrotic syndrome comprises **proteinuria, hypoalbuminaemia and oedema.** Glomerular abnormalities lead to excessive loss of protein in the urine, eventually of a severity such that the liver cannot synthesise proteins to keep pace. This leads to low protein levels in blood, particularly albumin. The oedema is an oncotic oedema due to the low serum albumin level.
A308. This glomerular disease is called **membranous nephropathy**.
A309. Membranous nephropathy has many precipitating factors, but in a man of this age, an underlying malignancy must be suspected.
See *Pathology*, p. 328.

A310. The lesion labelled **A** is an **epithelial crescent** derived from cells lining Bowman's capsule. The crescent proliferates rapidly and compresses the glomerular tuft out of existence, leading to rapidly progressive renal failure if enough glomeruli are affected.
A311. This is called **crescentic glomerulonephritis**.
A312. In this case the great majority of the glomeruli are affected, and the prognosis is poor, with little chance of spontaneous recovery of renal function. Prognosis is poor if more than 75% of glomeruli are affected by crescents.
A313. A number of diseases can produce crescentic glomerulonephritis, all appearing to have the common factor of severe destruction of glomerular capillary wall permitting leakage of blood into Bowman's space. In this case, the most likely disease is acute diffuse proliferative glomerulonephritis secondary to the viral infection. Note that the similar disease in children very rarely has this poor outcome.
See *Pathology*, p. 334.

A314. These nodules are Kimmelstiel–Wilson nodules.
A315. They are composed of nodular hyaline material, often concentrically laminated, derived from mesangial matrix.

A316. Diabetes mellitus.

A317. Glomerular effects are diffuse thickening of basement membrane, exudative lesions (fibrin caps) on glomerular capillary surface, diffuse mesangial matrix increase (diffuse diabetic glomerulosclerosis), and the nodules shown above. In addition, there is hyaline arterioloscerosis in pre-glomerular vessels, and a greatly increased predisposition to bacterial infection and papillary necrosis.
See *Pathology*, p. 335.

A318. The areas labelled **A** are the papillae of the renal medulla; they are abnormally pale due to necrosis—**renal papillary necrosis.**
A319. Papillary necrosis is frequently associated with:
 • Diabetic kidney disease.
 • Acute pyelonephritis.
 • Obstructive uropathy.
 • Chronic analgesic overdose (now rare).
A320. Papillary necrosis usually leads to acute renal failure, the necrotic papillae being shed and excreted in the urine.
See *Pathology*, p. 336.

A321. The high temperature and rigors indicate severe infection. The falling blood pressure and tachycardia indicate shock, in this instance of septicaemic origin.
A322. The small white dots are small cortical abscesses beneath the renal capsule. Similar abscesses would be seen scattered throughout cortex and medulla on the cut surface. The presence of abscesses in the kidney indicates **acute pyelonephritis.**
A323. Bacteria get into the kidney to produce pyelonephritis through two main routes:
 • **via the bloodstream** as part of a generalised septicaemia.
 • **ascending infection** from the lower urinary tract.
In most cases ascending infection is the cause.
See *Pathology*, p. 337.

A324. The kidneys are pale and show swelling—these features are typical of **acute tubular necrosis**.
A325. The proximal, distal and other tubules would show necrosis of their epithelial cells, many of which would have been shed. The interstitial space between the tubules would show oedema.
A326. Most cases are due to **hypovolaemia** or **prolonged hypotension**, often associated with massive blood loss, as in this case. Prolonged hypotension during emergency surgery may also have played a role.
A327. Some toxins can produce acute cortical necrosis: for example, ethylene glycol.
See *Pathology*, p. 339.

A328. The lesion labelled **A** is a large **renal adenocarcinoma** extending into perinephric fat; the variegated yellowish cut surface is characteristic. This tumour is derived from renal tubular epithelium.

A329. These malignant tumours enlarge and eventually break through the renal capsule into perinephric fat. They also invade renal vein tributaries, often growing as a solid core along the main renal vein at the kidney hilum. Bloodborne metastases are therefore common, with tendency to metastasise to lung, bone, brain, and occasionally unusual sites.
See *Pathology*, p. 341.

A330. The lesion is a malignant **nephroblastoma (Wilms' tumour)**, an embryonal tumour derived from primitive metanephros.

A331. Nephroblastoma is by far the most common malignant tumour which occurs in the kidney in children; its fleshy white cut surface is also characteristic.

A332. The behaviour and prognosis depend on two main factors: cytological differentiation and the extent of spread at the time of diagnosis. Even with extensive disseminated spread, there can be a high cure rate with a combination of radiotherapy and intensive chemotherapy, unless the tumour is very poorly differentiated histologically.
See *Pathology*, p. 343.

A333. Lesion **A** is a **papillary transitional cell carcinoma** of the bladder. It is a malignant lesion despite being apparently pedunculated.

A334. The smaller lesion is an identical transitional cell carcinoma arising from another part of the bladder wall. Transitional cell tumours of the urothelium are frequently multiple; for example, they may occur in the ureter or pelvicalyceal system of the kidney.

A335. Transitional cell tumours are graded histologically on the basis of cellular and nuclear pleomorphism and mitotic activity. The grading of a particular tumour relates to its biological behaviour. Staging of these tumours is based on the degree of bladder wall invasion and metastasis.

A336. This man's presenting symptom would have been **haematuria**, probably fresh blood.
See *Pathology*, p. 346.

A337. This kidney shows **adult polycystic disease** in which the functioning kidney is largely replaced by a mass of fluid-filled cysts. This is an **autosomal dominantly** inherited disease.

A338. The abnormal kidneys would have been palpable (and probably visible!) on examination of the abdomen. Laboratory investigation should have shown some degree of chronic renal failure.

A339. Although the cystic change begins in childhood, most patients present with slowly progressive chronic renal failure in adult life; they may also present with hypertension. The chronic renal failure is irreversible, and patients require chronic dialysis and renal transplantation. See *Pathology*, p. 348.

A340. The lesion is a **seminoma**, a malignant germ cell tumour of the testis.

A341. In a man of this age, seminoma is much the most likely testicular tumour; the other important tumours, teratoma and embryonal carcinoma, occur in a younger age group (17–30). In addition, the homogeneous creamy-white cut surface appearance, with no haemorrhage, necrosis or cysts, is characteristic.

A342. Seminoma initially metastasises via lymphatics to the lymph nodes around the iliac vessels and abdominal aorta. Only in the late stage does bloodstream spread occur. This is the basis of the treatment of this tumour—orchidectomy and irradiation of the lymph nodes around the iliac, arteries and abdominal aorta.
See *Pathology*, p. 354.

A343. The testis is replaced by a germ cell tumour of teratoma (embryonal carcinoma) type.

A344. Teratoma/embryonal carcinoma is much the most common tumour of the testis in a man of this age. In addition, the heterogeneous cut surface appearance, with numerous cysts, is characteristic of a tumour in the teratoma/embryonal carcinoma group. The precise classification of tumour type requires histological examination but, in general, the cystic areas (which are often lined by respiratory-type epithelium) are the more mature components of the teratoma, whereas the non-cystic fleshy areas are the less mature teratoma or embryonal carcinoma.

A345. In contrast to seminoma, the other important malignant germ cell tumours of the testis (teratoma/embryonal carcinoma), metastasise via the bloodstream at an early stage, the most common site for metastases being the lung and liver.

A346. Tumour cell markers are important in the diagnosis and management of testicular tumours; the most important markers are α-fetoprotein (AFP) and human chorionic gonadotropin (HCG), particularly in patients with non-seminomatous germ cell tumours. Raised serum levels of these markers in a patient with a testicular tumour usually indicates teratoma/embryonal carcinoma, and failure of the levels to return to normal after orchidectomy is an indication that there are metastatic tumour deposits. Similarly, elevation of the serum level of markers after initial treatment indicates the development of metastases, an indication for further chemotherapy.
See *Pathology*, p. 356.

A347. Structure **A** is the grossly distorted and compressed prostatic urethra. Such severe distortion and compression would have interfered with the passage of urine, which is responsible for the patient's most likely presenting symptom: **difficulty in micturition**, with probable chronic retention of urine.

A348. The disease is **benign prostatic hyperplasia**, which is very common in men over the age of 70. The periurethral prostatic glands undergo nodular hyperplasia, and **B** indicates one of the larger hyperplastic nodules.

A349. The prostate gland can be palpated through the anterior wall of the rectum on **rectal examination**. Benign prostatic enlargement such as this is usually felt as a smooth rubbery enlargement, in contrast to malignant enlargement of the prostate which is hard, craggy and irregular.

See *Pathology*, p. 359.

A350. Adenocarcinoma of the prostate; the example shown is well differentiated, with close resemblance to normal prostatic glands.

A351. The presence of **osteosclerotic deposits** in vertebral bodies pointed to the prostate gland, since prostatic carcinoma is one of the few tumours which produce osteosclerotic metastases as opposed to osteolytic deposits, the more common pattern of metastatic carcinoma in bone.

A352. The needle was introduced into the periphery of the prostate gland through the anterior rectal wall. Carcinoma of the prostate begins in the outer prostatic glands, and per-urethral prostatic biopsy may miss the tumour.

A353. Prostatic carcinoma spreads locally to invade the bladder, by lymphatics to pelvic and para-aortic nodes, and by the bloodstream, particularly to bones of the vertebra and pelvis. Raised serum levels of prostate-specific antigen and acid phosphatase may indicate metastatic disease.

See *Pathology*, p. 359.

A354. The abnormality is an exophytic growth in the lower half of the right labium majus, with some deep infiltration into the more lateral skin. The tumour is a well-differentiated squamous cell carcinoma of the vulva, of verrucous type.

A355. This particular pattern of squamous carcinoma is slow growing, exophytic, but invades locally. Lymph node metastasis is rare and usually occurs only in neglected lesions which present late where there is very extensive local invasion (as in this case).

A356. Squamous carcinoma of the vulva in general occurs in elderly women, and the verrucous pattern is largely confined to old women. However, non-invasive malignancy of the vulva, **vulval intraepithelial neoplasia** (**VIN**), can occur in younger women, and may be associated with human papilloma virus (HPV) infection of vulval epithelium.

A357. Superficial inguinal lymph nodes, which is where lymph node metastases first occur.
See *Pathology*, p. 362.

A358. The epithelium on the left is normal ectocervical epithelium, that on the right is abnormal.
A359. The abnormal epithelium shows severe dysplastic change, with loss of the normal stratified pattern; the squamous epithelial cells with large abnormal nuclei extend to the epithelial surface.
A360. This is **cervical intraepithelial neoplasia (CIN)**, of a severe degree. It may be diagnosed by cytological examination of a cervical smear when the abnormal dysplastic epithelial cells (which are easily shed—see arrows) can be identified. Further support comes from colposcopic biopsy of abnormal areas of cervical epithelium.
A361. The major risk is the potential for progression to invasive carcinoma of the cervix within 10–15 years.
See *Pathology*, p. 366.

A362. The lesion is a large endometrial adenocarcinoma distending the endometrial cavity and invading the myometrium almost to the serosal surface at the uterine fundus.
A363. By histological examination of endometrial curettings.
A364. In the early stages the tumour spreads by local invasion through the myometrial wall and down into cervix, later followed by spread outside the uterus into pelvic tissues, including bladder and rectum. Spread by the lymphatics and the bloodstream can lead to both local (e.g. vaginal) and distant metastases, particularly para-aortic nodes.
See *Pathology*, p. 373.

A365. They are benign leiomyomas of the myometrium ('fibroids').
A366. Multiple leiomyomas distort the uterus and increase the size of the endometrial lining surface, thus providing a greater amount of endometrium to be shed at menstruation. Sometimes, as in the central lower oval fibroid in this picture, the lesions are submucosal, protruding into the endometrial cavity, again increasing the extent of the endometrium.
A367. The lesions grow slowly until the menopause, after which they slowly regress, being dependent on oestrogen stimulation for their growth. If they do not present because of menstrual irregularities, they may present during pregnancy, sometimes inducing spontaneous abortion and premature or obstructed labour. Sometimes they present as a large lower abdominal mass, occasionally producing urinary symptoms because of pressure on the bladder.
See *Pathology*, p. 375.

A368. The organ is the right Fallopian tube.

A369. The abnormality is heavy bleeding into the Fallopian tube due to the presence of a **tubal ectopic pregnancy**.

A370. Her abnormal vital signs indicate shock, and are the result of acute blood loss into both the Fallopian tube and also into the peritoneal cavity: ectopic pregnancies frequently erode through the wall of the Fallopian tube, permitting bleeding into the peritoneal cavity.

A371. There is often an underlying structural abnormality of the Fallopian tube: the most common abnormalities are scarring secondary to previous episodes of infection (salpingitis) or previous tubal surgery.

See *Pathology*, p. 383.

A372. The disease is **fibrocystic disease of the breast ('fibroadenosis')**.

A373. A indicates one of the important components of this growth disorder, a cyst lined by apocrine-type epithelium. Cysts are a prominent feature, increasing in incidence with the approach of the menopause.

A374. The main components of this disease are:
- Increase in fibrous tissue.
- Proliferation of the epithelium of the breast lobule ('adenosis').
- Cystic dilatation of ducts, often with apocrine metaplasia.

A375. 10% of all women have clinically apparent lumpiness in the breast due to this common disease, but histological examination reveals minor degrees of the change in up to 40% of women.

See *Pathology*, p. 388.

A376. The lesion is most likely to be a **fibroadenoma** on clinical grounds; this is the most common cause of a solitary rounded rubbery lump in the breast in a young woman. The histology confirms the diagnosis: **A** is the epithelial ('adenoma') component and **B** being the proliferating stromal ('fibro-') component.

A377. It is completely benign.

See *Pathology*, p. 390.

A378. The lesion labelled **A** is an **invasive adenocarcinoma of the breast**.

A379. The nipple retraction is due to invasion by tumour. Invasion of overlying breast skin frequently leads to dimpling in tumours which arise near the surface.

A380. Most invasive carcinomas of the breast excite a vigorous fibrous stromal reaction, the fibrous tissue being responsible for the hardness of the lesion on palpation.

A381. Invasive breast cancer spreads via lymphatics, usually to lymph nodes in the axilla, and via the bloodstream, particularly to

the lungs and pleura, bones and liver. Blood-borne metastasis may become manifest many years after apparently successful surgical and radiotherapy treatment of the primary tumour.
See *Pathology*, p. 393.

A382. The original red area in the nipple was **Paget's disease of the nipple.**
A383. She required mastectomy because of the underlying invasive ductal carcinoma.
A384. Paget's disease is caused by breast carcinoma cells that spread along the mammary and nipple ducts, emerge on the surface and invade the epidermis. The underlying breast tumour is usually of the ductal type and may be either intraduct or invasive. The adenocarcinoma cells within the nipple skin are larger and paler than the epidermal cells and are called Paget cells.
See *Pathology*, p. 394.

A385. A indicates a recent cerebral infarct; **B** indicates an old cystic and gliotic cavity that results from an old infarct.
A386. The brain on the left came from the patient who died shortly after onset of hemiplegia; the brain on the right is from the patient who survived for 2 years. In the intervening time the infarcted area of brain has undergone liquefactive necrosis with reactive gliosis.
A387. Both infarcts are in the vascular territory supplied by the middle cerebral artery on that side.
A388. Both lesions have been caused by occlusion of the main middle cerebral artery: either by **thrombosis**, forming on atheroma; or by **embolus**—for example, from thrombosis in the left side of the heart or from a narrowed carotid artery in the neck.
See *Pathology*, p. 402.

A389. The lesion is a large haematoma due to massive intracerebral haemorrhage, with rupture into the ventricles.
A390. The lesion has originated in the basal ganglia region, the most common site for intracerebral haemorrhage.
A391. The patient probably suffered from systemic hypertension, hypertensive vascular damage being the most common cause of cerebral haemorrhage.
A392. The basal ganglia region is the most common site for hypertensive cerebral haemorrhage, because prolonged hypertension produces hyaline arteriosclerosis and small micro-aneurysms (Charcot–Bouchard aneurysms) in the fine perforating vessels (lenticulo-striate vessels) running from the middle cerebral artery to the basal ganglia region. Haemorrhage is due to rupture of these abnormal vessels.
See *Pathology*, p. 404.

A393. The brain shows a recent subarachnoid haemorrhage extending over the base of the brain, mainly the cerebellum.

A394. The commonest cause of subarachnoid haemorrhage is rupture of a small spherical aneurysm in the vessels of the circle of Willis. These are called berry aneurysms, and are mainly seen where the carotid bifurcates into middle (**C**) and anterior (**A**) cerebral arteries. The aneurysms here (**B**) are at the origin of the left middle cerebral artery. Less commonly, berry aneurysms arise near the origin of the posterior cerebral artery (**D**), as a result of developmental defects in the internal elastic lamina of the cerebral arteries.

A395. Cerebrospinal fluid (obtained by lumbar puncture) shows blood staining. The haemorrhage can usually be visualised by imaging, which also shows its precise location and severity.
See *Pathology*, p. 404, 400.

A396. The lesion labelled **A** is an extensive area ('plaque') of demyelination alongside the lateral ventricle, a typical site for large lesions.

A397. The patient suffered from **multiple sclerosis**, which is a primary demyelinating disease.

A398. Yes, as its name implies, multiple sclerosis is associated with multiple areas of demyelination in the white matter.
See *Pathology*, p. 414.

A399. The cerebral hemisphere in the abnormal brain is greatly reduced in size as a result of loss of both grey matter and white matter; the brain shows **cerebral atrophy**.

A400. The region identified by the label **A** is the hippocampal region. Compare it with the equivalent area in the normal brain; it is the area which shows the most marked atrophy in many types of dementia and relates to memory loss.

A401. The most likely cause of this patient's dementia is **Alzheimer's disease**, which is the most common neurodegenerative disorder manifesting as dementia.
See *Pathology*, p. 416.

A402. The lesion in (b) is **spina bifida occulta.** Failure of development of the bony arch of the spinal column is often associated with a skin dimple, sinus track or subcutaneous lipoma.

A403. The lesion in (c) is a **meningocele.** In addition to the bony arch defect, the meninges pouch out as far as the surface of the skin. The spinal cord may be normal or abnormal.

A404. The lesion in (d) is a **meningomyelocele**. There is failure of bony arch formation, and pouching of the meninges and abnormal spinal cord which protrude above the skin level as a cystic mass.

A405. Damage to the spinal cord and nerve roots leads to paraplegia, urinary and faecal incontinence and lower limb deformities; the urinary problems frequently lead to chronic renal failure because of recurrent infection. The severe degrees of neural-tube defect may be associated with the Arnold–Chiari malformation, in which the cerebellum tonsils extend into the foramen magnum associated with the hydrocephalus.
See *Pathology*, p. 420.

A406. The slow-growing, low-grade astrocytoma tumour is indicated by **A**; the highly malignant, rapidly growing glial tumour is indicated by **B**.
A407. Low-grade astrocytomas appear as ill-defined pale areas, sometimes with focal softening, which seem to blend into adjacent normal brain. The most highly malignant glial tumours, glioblastoma (**B**), grow rapidly and often form haemorrhagic masses with necrosis.
A408. The two types of glioma illustrated are the opposite extremes of a continuum with varying degrees of differentiation. The low-grade astrocytomas (**A**) are associated with many years' survival, although surgical removal is difficult because of poor delineation from normal brain. Glioblastomas, however, have a median survival of about 10 months from the time of diagnosis, usually causing death by rapid local growth, brain destruction and haemorrhage.
See *Pathology*, p. 424, 425.

A409. The lesion is a **nodular malignant melanoma of the skin**.
A410. The flat lesion was probably a **superficial spreading malignant melanoma**, and the nodular malignant melanoma has developed within it.
A411. The development of nodular malignant melanoma makes this a poor prognosis tumour, with a high likelihood of metastatic spread. Had the lesion been excised when it was a flat superficial spreading malignant melanoma, the prognosis would have been considerably better, with less chance of metastatic spread.
A412. Initial spread is by lymphatics to regional lymph nodes: in this case, the inguinal lymph nodes. Sometimes, clumps of tumour cells are trapped in lymphatics on the way to the lymph node, producing multiple satellite metastases in the skin and subcutis.
See *Pathology*, p. 467.

A413. This is called a '**pyogenic granuloma**' and is composed of a proliferating mass of vascular granulation tissue containing numerous inflammatory cells. There is often surface ulceration.
A414. A frequent precipitating factor on the finger is a penetrating injury—in this case, due to a rose thorn.
A415. Young pregnant women develop pyogenic granulomas in the mouth, particularly in gingival mucosa.
see *Pathology*, p. 470.

A416. The disease is **osteomalacia**, in which there is defective mineralisation of bone osteoid; this leads to soft bone, with predisposition to bone pain, fractures and bone distortion.

A417. Osteomalacia is usually the result of **vitamin D deficiency**, which may be due to either inadequate dietary intake (now rare) or inadequate endogenous synthesis of vitamin D (vitamin D is normally synthesised from a skin precursor, the active metabolites being produced in the liver and kidney). Osteomalacia may sometimes result from a chronic renal disease (due to failure of production of active vitamin D metabolite) or from malabsorption states (where there is inadequate absorption of dietary vitamin D and calcium).

A418. Although in this woman there may be a dietary factor, particularly if she is an extreme vegan, the most likely cause is inadequate body synthesis of vitamin D in the skin because of extensive covering of the skin for social and cultural reasons in women from the Indian subcontinent.
See *Pathology*, p. 478.

A419. The lesion at the lower end of the femur is a large **osteosarcoma**, a malignant tumour of osteoblasts. It has arisen in the medullary cavity close to the metaphyseal plate near the bone end and has spread extensively in the marrow cavity, breaking through cortical bone into the surrounding soft tissue.

A420. These are highly malignant tumours which grow rapidly and metastasise early via the bloodstream with extensive bloodborne metastases, particularly in the lung.

A421. Yes. These commonly occur in adolescent children, more often in boys than in girls; the bones around the knee, either the lower end of the femur or the upper end of the tibia, are the most common sites. The tumour does not commonly occur in adults, except as a rare complication of long-standing active Paget's disease in the elderly.
See *Pathology*, p. 485.

A422. The photograph at the top shows typical changes in the hand in **osteoarthritis**; the picture at the bottom shows the changes in typical long-standing **rheumatoid arthritis**. The osteoarthritic hand is characterised by the presence of hard nodular swellings on the joints of the fingers (Heberden's nodes). The hand affected by long-standing rheumatoid arthrtitis shows disproportionate enlargement of the knuckles, characteristic ulnar deviation, and marked atrophy of the muscles of the hand.

A423. Osteoarthritis is a degenerative disease which occurs in joints that are constantly exposed to wear and tear, and may (as in this former typist) be partly occupational. It may also occur as a secondary change in a joint previously damaged by trauma or some

other joint disease, e.g. gout. **Rheumatoid arthritis** is a systemic autoimmune disease, associated with the presence of a circulating autoantibody, which particularly affects the joints. It is the most important type of 'seropositive arthritis'.
See *Pathology*, p. 489, 491.

A424. The diagnosis is gout, a crystal arthritis due to excess deposition of urate; the metatarsophalangeal of the big toe is a typical site.

A425. Although most patients with gout have some form or history of an acute arthritis, some patients present as a chronic arthritis. Deposits of urate crystals in the subcutaneous tissue may present as visible and palpable nodules filled with white chalky material, which is the insoluble urate ('gouty tophi').

A426. The local complications are:
• chronic osteoarthritis occurring in the joint previously damaged by gout.
• masses of urate around the joint eroding the skin and discharging chalky material.

The systemic complications are:
• interstitial nephritis due to urate crystal deposition in the kidney.
• renal calculus formation, the stones being composed largely of urate.

See *Pathology*, p. 492.